Keto Meal Prep 2019

A Step by Step 30-Days Meal Prep Guide to Make Delicious and Easy Ketogenic Recipes for a Rapid Weight Loss

Stefano Villa

© **Copyright 2019 - All rights reserved – Stefano Villa.**

The content contained within this book may not be reproduced, duplicated or transmitted without direct written permission from the author or the publisher.

Under no circumstances will any blame or legal responsibility be held against the publisher, or author, for any damages, reparation, or monetary loss due to the information contained within this book. Either directly or indirectly.

Legal Notice:

This book is copyright protected. This book is only for personal use. You cannot amend, distribute, sell, use, quote or paraphrase any part, or the content within this book, without the consent of the author or publisher.

Disclaimer Notice:

Please note the information contained within this document is for educational and entertainment purposes only. All effort has been executed to present accurate, up to date, and reliable, complete information. No warranties of any kind are declared or implied. Readers acknowledge that the author is not engaging in the rendering of legal, financial, medical or professional advice. The content within this book has been derived from various sources. Please consult a licensed professional before attempting any techniques outlined in this book.

By reading this document, the reader agrees that under no circumstances is the author responsible for any losses, direct or indirect, which are incurred as a result of the use of information contained within this document, including, but not limited to, — errors, omissions, or inaccuracies.

Table of Contents

Introduction 6
Chapter 1. Ketosis Explained 8
   Making Fat Burning as Beneficial as Possible 8
   Ketones Provide Energy for the Brain 9
   Are Carbohydrates Needed by the Brain? 9
   Benefits of Ketosis 10
Chapter 2. Ketogenic Diet 16
   What is the Ketogenic Diet? 16
   Working Out Your Macronutrient Ratio 17
   Why Do You Need to Start a Ketogenic Diet? 19
   What to Eat and What Not to Eat 21
Chapter 3. Disadvantages of a Ketogenic Diet 25
   Hypoglycemia 26
   HPA Axis Dysregulation 29
   Keto Breath 34
   Precautions for Certain Situations 35
   Exogenous Ketones 36
Chapter 4. Starting a Ketogenic Diet 38
   Who Should Start a Ketogenic Diet Plan? 38
   10 Things To Do To Combat Keto Flu Toxins During The 28 Days 41
Chapter 5. How to Get Started 46
   Tips for going out days 47
Chapter 6. 28-Day Diet Plan 54
   Week 1 54
   Week 2 65
   Week 3 74
   Week 4 82
Chapter 7. Ketogenic Diet Recipes 91
   Almond Lemon Cake Sandwiches 91
   Inside Out Bacon Burger 94

Bacon & Mozzarella Meatballs 96
Bacon Infused Sugar Snap Peas 98
BBQ Pulled Chicken 99
Buffalo Chicken Strips 101
Bulletproof Coffee 103
Chai Spice Mug Cake 104
Bacon Cheddar Explosion 106
Cheddar Chorizo Meatballs 108
Cheesy Scrambled Eggs 110
Cheesy Spinach 111
Chicken Roulade 112
Buffalo Chicken Strip Slider 114
Bacon, Cheddar & Chive Mug Biscuit 116
Orange & Cinnamon Beef Stew 118
Coffee & Red Wine Beef Stew 120
Crispy Curry Rubbed Chicken Thigh 122
Drunken Five Spice Beef 124
Cheesy Frittata Muffins 126
Fried Queso Fresco 128
Lemon Rosemary Chicken 129
Keto Szechuan Chicken 131
Not Your Caveman's Chili 133
Omnivore Burger with Roasted Almonds & Creamed Spinach 135
Bacon Wrapped Pork Tenderloin 137
Red Pepper Spinach Salad 139
Roasted Pecan Green Beans 140
Shrimp & Cauliflower Curry 142
Simple Lunch Salad 145
Keto Snickerdoodle Cookies 146
Low Carb Spice Cakes 148
Chicken and Bacon Sausage Stir Fry 150
Taco Tartlets 152
Thai Peanut Chicken 155

- Vanilla Latte Cookies 157
- Vegetable Medley 159
- Chapter 8. Ketogenic Smoothie Recipes 161
  - Shopping List 161
  - Chocolate Almond Smoothie 163
  - Pumpkin Pie Smoothie 164
  - Green Smoothie 165
  - Honeydew and Avocado Smoothie 166
  - Carrot Asparagus Green Smoothie 168
  - Avocado Raspberry Smoothie 169
  - Triple Green Smoothie 170
  - Almond Berry Smoothie 171
  - Kale and Brazil Nut Smoothie 173
  - Calming Cucumber Smoothie 174
  - Spiced Cashew Butter Smoothie 175
  - Spiced Chocolate Smoothie 177
  - Orange Coconut Smoothie 179
  - Banana-Lettuce Smoothie 180
- Keto-Friendly Snacks 182
- Chapter 9. Ketogenic Diet Success Tips 183
  - Tips and Tricks for Maintaining the Diet 183
  - Planning Meals for Long-Term Success 187
- Chapter 10. FAQ 189
- Conclusion 203
- Sources 204

Introduction

It's possible that you have been informed for years or even decades to consume a great amount of whole-grain carbohydrates and stay away from saturated fat at all costs — fat is, however, not bad for you. Fat, maybe saturated fat especially even helps your body run like a well-oiled machine would. The ketogenic diet's basis is the human body's need for fat, which encourages that as an individual you should obtain a large portion of your calories—about 75 percent—from fat and just 5 to 10 percent from carbohydrates. The rest of the calories are obtained from proteins of high-quality.

The ketogenic diet is neither a novel trend nor is it a fad diet. Actually, it's been available for decades. In the 1920s, it was utilized as the main method of treatment for hard-to-control epilepsy in young kids—and it was remarkably efficient. It eventually fell out of fashion with the increasing presence of anti-seizure drugs. Even if that fix implied the potential for more side effects, individuals preferred a quick solution. Individuals following nutritional ketogenic diets today report weight reduction, increased energy levels, better mood, enhanced concentration, and mental clarity.

Nevertheless, mainstream press and even a few healthcare experts tend to present the ketogenic diet in a negative light. Just like fat, ketones, which are compounds made when the body starts to utilize fat in place of carbohydrates for energy, do not have a good reputation. Majority of the worries surrounding ketones and the ketogenic diet are unwarranted or are a consequence of confusion between the two terms "ketosis" and "ketoacidosis."

This confusion and assumptions about the ketogenic diet—like the idea that all types of fat are bad for you—might be "presenting barriers that are not necessary to their use as therapeutic tools in the hand of the physician" as stated by the European Journal of Clinical Nutrition

At this point let us put the rumors to rest and understand why fat is not only good but is basic to the maintenance of optimal health. Actually, sugar, carbohydrates, and processed vegetable oils are responsible for weight gain and the increasing incidence of chronic health conditions to a great extent. Carbohydrates limitation and replacement with both saturated and unsaturated fats—the ketogenic diet's basis—is not only capable of helping you lose weight, but it can also help you remain healthy for years to come.

Chapter 1. Ketosis Explained

'Keto,' from the word ketosis, is made from Ketones, the term for the body's energy molecules. This is a second source of energy for the body that is utilized when glucose (blood sugar) is insufficient to meet the body's needs. Ketones are generated when the number of carbohydrates (the major source of glucose) consumed is very little, in combination to a limited amount of protein (additional protein is converted into glucose.) Under these conditions, the liver converts fat to ketones which are then transported into the bloodstream. The body cells use this as a source of energy, like glucose. They can also be utilized by the brain. This is essential, as the brain cannot get its energy directly from fat, and it is a rapid energy-consuming organ.

Making Fat Burning as Beneficial as Possible

There are two ways of achieving Ketosis; the first way is to consume a ketogenic diet. The other is to begin a period of fasting.

Under these conditions, immediately the body's restricted stores of glucose are being depleted, the whole body changes its source of energy supply to fat almost completely. The quantity of insulin (the fat accumulating hormone) becomes reduced, and fat is rapidly used up. Thus, your fat reserves are easily accessible and can easily be consumed. This is excellent for shedding off excess weight. Research has proven that the ketogenic diet produced greater weight loss, faster. There are many other additional benefits. The condition where the body generates sufficient ketones to add up to high levels in the blood (greater than 0.5mM) is referred to as ketosis. The most rapid way to achieve ketosis is through fasting- not consuming any food at all- but that is impossible to do forever.

However, a rigorous 'keto' or low-carb diet can be consumed for unlimited periods of time. It also produces ketosis. The results produced are as beneficial as those produced by fasting (like weight loss) without necessarily fasting.

Ketones Provide Energy for the Brain

There is a popular erroneous belief that the brain requires carbs. In truth, the brain gladly uses up carbs when you consume them; yet if you don't consume enough carbs, the brain is equally glad to burn ketones instead.

Are Carbohydrates Needed by the Brain?

This is one of the brain's most essential functions for basic survival. Since the body can only store carbs for one or two days, the brain would completely stop functioning after going without food for a couple of days. Or, it would rapidly have to convert protein in the muscle into glucose – a very inadequate process, just to ensure that the brain keeps functioning. This would make us emaciated rapidly. It would also have resulted in the extinction of the human race before we had food available 24/7.

Luckily, the evolution of our bodies has made it smarter than that. Usually, we have long lasting fat reserves to enable us to survive for many weeks (probably months) without food. The body makes sure that the brain can function by using these fat stores via ketosis.

A lot of people are more energized and can concentrate more when the source of energy for the brain is ketones. And it definitely makes fat loss easier, assuming you are trying to lose weight.

Benefits of Ketosis

A ketogenic diet enables you to eat some of your favorite foods like eggs, bacon, butter, steak and also allows you to improve your health and prevent chronic illnesses by being in a condition of nutritional ketosis.

Ketosis aides healthy weight loss

When people are about to begin a new diet regimen, their most important concern is losing weight. And if you are like every other person, you already know that the low-fat diet your doctor has consistently recommended for years only increases your 'fat reserves' instead of depleting it.

Is ketogenic diet really the solution to all your weight loss problems? Though, contrary to what common sense may suggest, consuming a diet rich in fat can help you burn fat and lose excess weight!

Ketosis speeds up metabolism. Limiting Carb intake can increase the total amount of energy expended because it is more expensive to generate ketones from fat than to convert carbs and protein into glucose. Although ketones are a more effective source of fuel, the process of producing them increases your metabolism.

Ketosis reduces insulin - the fat storing hormone. Even if you are not diabetic, it is possible you are prediabetic, this means that sometimes your insulin levels are habitually elevated. And if you have no previous knowledge, if your insulin levels are always elevated, then it would've difficult for you to lose weight, irrespective of how much you exercise or how rigorously you limit your caloric intake.

Luckily, the ketogenic diet has been proven to be effective in treating insulin resistance by enhancing insulin sensitivity. Eventually, the more improved your insulin sensitivity, the less effort is required to lose weight

Ketosis controls hunger. It takes a longer period of time for fat to be digested than carbohydrates, consuming a meal majorly consisting of fat means that you will feel satiated for a longer period of time. The advantage of this long-lasting satiety so that you won't need to constantly consume snacks, allowing you to restrict your calories without even counting.

Ketosis enhances mental and cognitive health
A lot of us are still in a haze of confusion, trying to force our brains into concentrating while fighting anxiety and depression. Instead of using yet another prescription pill, have you considered the advantages of ketosis for your mental and cognitive performance?

Ketosis improves memory. In contrast to popular beliefs, memory loss is necessarily not a normal part of aging. In fact, a lot of people that have poor or spotty memory are not really old. Luckily, ketosis can enhance memory. The greater the number of Ketones in blood, the better the improvement in memory.

Ketosis helps to stabilize moods. Ketosis may be beneficial in stabilizing the mood of people who have bipolar disorder. A few of the extracellular changes usually observed in ketosis is likely to reduce intracellular sodium concentrations, an important quality of all effective mood stabilizing medications.

Ketosis improves focus. Have you ever been under the pressure of an impending deadline, only for you to start surfing through the web rather than focusing on your work? Although, we realize that our work should have the greatest priority, concentrating long enough to get it done can prove to be very difficult.

And if you are still unable to concentrate, it is possible that you have an inadequate amount of neurotransmitters- GABA and glutamate, but entering into a ketogenic state will help your body even out these two neurotransmitters. Proper balance results in improved concentration, while decreasing stress and worry.

Ketosis decreases inflammatory reactions in the brain. It is well known that the joints and muscles can be inflamed; but, do you realize that the brain can also be affected? In fact, your terrible moods and cognitive problems could just be another symptom of an inflammatory reaction in the brain. Here are some red flags that something is going on in your brain

- Symptoms of an inflamed brain
- Concentration problems

- Groggy brain
- Stuttering or stammering when speaking
- Psychosis and mood disorders
- Depression
- Poor memory

Luckily, ketosis can stop inflammation in the brain by providing a substantial amount of antioxidant protection that helps fight against oxidants that destroy body cells that causes depression and poor memory.

Ketosis prevents and manages chronic illnesses

In spite of the widespread fact that the ketogenic diet is the best solution for weight loss, would you believe that nutritional ketosis was primarily developed to treat children who have epilepsy?

As a matter of fact, the ketogenic diet is gradually getting known for being an effective treatment for a number of chronic, debilitating illnesses that were treated exclusively with medications in the past!

Type 2 Diabetes. For someone with Type 2 Diabetes, you know how annoying it can be to regularly monitor your insulin levels, following your Carb intake and be constantly worried about the long-term effect of elevated insulin levels on your health.

Luckily, by following a ketogenic diet plan; it is possible to reverse insulin insensitivity. As a matter of fact, a diet rich in fat and low in carbs has been proven to enhance insulin sensitivity by 75 percent.

Research and shown that following a strict ketogenic diet plan can also help you stop taking your diabetic medication altogether.

Heart Diseases. With higher than normal levels of cholesterol and familial history of heart disease, you may initially assume that the ketogenic diet would be the most unsuitable diet plan for a healthy heart.

Though, initially, it may seem paradoxical, consuming carbs in excess is the main cause of increased levels of triglycerides, particularly the consumption of fructose (as seen in corn syrup rich in fructose). On the other hand, a ketogenic diet reduces LDL cholesterol (the harmful cholesterol) while elevating HDL cholesterol (the helpful cholesterol). So when a person lets go of carbs, it is likely that there will be a high reduction in their blood triglyceride. And since increased triglycerides indicate heart disease, reducing levels of triglycerides is important towards lowering the risking experiencing heart attack or a stroke.

Cancer. Adopting the ketogenic diet plan helps treat and control cancer. Definitely, it is important that you speak with your doctor prior to beginning a new diet when you have cancer; but, recent studies have proved the beneficial effects that this diet provided by reducing cancerous cells and shrinking the size of tumors.

A ketogenic diet efficiently manages cancer because you are depriving cancer cells of their most preferred food – sugar. Cancer cells are not the same as normal cells because they have ten times more insulin receptors that transport sugar into the cell. In summary, cancer cells need sugar to survive, and they grow when you consume a diet rich in sugar.

As an advantage, cancer cells are destroyed so they can't efficiently use fats as a source of energy. So when you consume a low-carb, high-fat diet, you are depriving the cancer cells while nourishing your own healthy cells.

Chapter 2. Ketogenic Diet

Since you now have a thorough comprehension of how the body gets energy and what ketosis entails (a state where fuel comes from fat instead of carbohydrates), it is time to start using all these information. From the name, it can be deduced that the ketogenic diet is a diet regimen that exerts your body's natural intelligence by driving your body into a state of ketosis. Innately, your body already knows how to do this when you do not consume carbohydrates, but the objective of the ketogenic diet is to forcefully enable this and to make it continue for as long as you need it to.

What is the Ketogenic Diet?

When on the ketogenic diet, the majority of your calories come from fat, and you consume carbohydrates only sparingly. Contrary to a typical low-carbohydrate diet, the ketogenic diet is not a high-protein diet; it is a moderate-protein, low-carbohydrate, and high-fat diet. However, your actual macronutrient ratio depends on your individual requirements. This is an example of a nutritional Ketogenic diet:

- Protein: 15 to 30 percent of total calories.

- Fat: 60 to 70 percent of total calories

- Carbohydrate: 5 to 10 percent of total calories.

These are just universal principles, but most people on an effective ketogenic diet use this rough estimate. You will have to work out your individual macronutrient ratios, so you can be able to estimate the number of calories to be consumed. As you continue your diet and your body begins to look different, you might be required to calculate these numbers again and adjust it to suit your diet regimen.

Working Out Your Macronutrient Ratio
To calculate your macronutrient ratio, you must first calculate how many calories you have to consume. Many online calculators can help you with this, but to do it by yourself, you use a formula known as the Mifflin-St Jeor formula which is written as:
- Men: 10*weight (kg) +6.25 * height(cm) -5 * age (years) +5
- Women: 10 * weight (kg) +6.25 * height (cm) -5* age (years) -161

To make this easier to understand, let's us use the formula for a 30-year-old, 160 pounds (72.7kg) woman who is 5 feet 5 inches (165.1cm) tall. When you insert this woman's data into the Mifflin-St Jeor formula, the resulting number of calories to be consumed is 1,448 calories each day. Now, using the estimated macronutrient percentages, work out the number of nutrients she needs to eat in order to follow an effective ketogenic diet regimen.

Carbohydrates
When on a ketogenic diet, carbohydrates should make up just 5 to 10 percent of the calories consumed. Most people on the ketogenic diet remain at the lower limit of 5 percent, but the actual amount required is dependent on your body. Sadly, there is no universal approach to this; you have to keep experimenting until you find a solution. You could choose a percentage that makes you comfortable and try that for a few weeks. If the results are not to your liking, you will have to tweak the nutrient ratios and calculate them again. Obtaining 7

percent of your calories from carbohydrates is preferable to start with.

To work out how many grams of carbohydrates this is; using the previous example of 1,448 calories, multiply that by 7 then divide by 4 (as 1 gram of carbohydrates contains 4 calories). The remaining number is the number of carbs in grams that you should consume each day. In this instance, the number is 25 grams.

Total Carb vs. Net Carb

When calculating carb on a ketogenic diet, Net Carb is the focus, instead of Total Carb. Net Carb is the quantity of Carb remaining after subtracting the amounting fiber (in grams) from Total Carb (in grams). For example of a food item contains 10 grams of carbs but 7 grams is from fiber, the total quantity of net carb is 3 grams. You can calculate the 3 grams as your total each day, instead of the 10 grams.

Fat

After calculating carbs, continue with fat. Here too, the particular amount you will require is dependent on your individual requirement; Although, getting 75 percent of your calories from fat is nice, to begin with. To calculate the quantity of fat required in grams, still using the previous example of 1,448 calories, multiply this by 75 and divide the value gotten by 9 (1 gram of fat is equal to 9 calories) The number remaining is the total amount of fat needed to the day. In this instance, 121 grams.

Proteins

Calculating proteins is not as difficult after calculating carbs and fat. The remaining calories which is 18 percent should be from protein. To calculate this amount on grams, multiply the total amount of calories (1,448) by 18 and divide the result gotten by 4 (as 1 gram of protein is equal to 4 calories). The number remaining is the total amount of protein required for the day. In this instance, 65 grams.

Why Do You Need to Start a Ketogenic Diet?

The benefits of being on a ketogenic diet are endless. From weight loss and elevated energy levels to therapeutic medical uses. Almost everyone can profit from consuming a low-carb, high-fat diet. Below are some of the advantages of being on a ketogenic diet.

1. Weight loss. The ketogenic diet simply uses body fat as a source of fuel- so there is visible weight loss. While on a ketogenic diet, the levels of your insulin drastically decrease which makes your body a fat consuming machine.

With scientific research, the results of a ketogenic diet have been proven to be better when compared to low-fat, high-carb diets even in the long run. A number of people include MCT oil in their diet by drinking keto-proof coffee in the morning (MCT oil boosts ketone generation and fat loss).

2. Control blood sugar. Naturally, keto reduces levels of blood glucose as a result of the type of foods consumed. Research has shown that the ketogenic diet is more effectual on controlling and preventing diabetes as compared to low-calorie diets.

If you are prediabetic or a Type 2 Diabetic, you should think about starting a ketogenic diet.

3. Mental performance. A lot of people particularly use the ketogenic diet because it enhances mental performance. Ketones are an excellent source of brain fuel; when you reduce your Carb consumption, you prevent large increases in blood sugar. Together, this results in better concentration and focus

Research has shown that increased consumption of fatty acids can positively enhance our brain function.

4. Increased energy and normalized hunger. By providing your body with a more suitable and dependable source of energy, you will feel more revitalized during the day. Fats have been proven to be the most efficient molecule to consume as fuel. Additionally, fat provides more nourishment and leaves you in a 'full' (satiated) state for a longer time

5. Epilepsy. Since the early 1900s, the ketogenic diet has been effectively utilized to treat epilepsy. It is one of the most commonly used therapies for children with poorly controlled epilepsy today. One of the major benefits of the ketogenic diet and epilepsy is that only a few medications are used and it is still properly controlled. In recent years, studies have shown impressive outcomes in adults treated with Keto too.

6. Cholesterol and blood pressure. A ketogenic diet has been proven to reduce the levels of cholesterol and triglyceride which have been shown to be associated with accumulation in the arteries. Particularly, low-carb, high-fat diets show a startling increase in HDL and reduction in LDL particle when compared with low-fat diets. Researches done on low-carb diets have shown that blood pressure is improved with the ketogenic diet as compared to other diets.

Excess weight is responsible for some blood pressure problems, and this is an additional benefit as keto results in weight loss. If your blood pressure is high or you have other related problems with your blood pressure, you can learn to use Keto to lower your blood pressure here

7. Insulin resistance. Type 2 Diabetes can develop as a result of poorly managed insulin resistance. Research has shown that a low-carb, ketogenic diet helps people reduce insulin levels to healthy ranges.

Even if you are an athlete, you can profit from maximizing insulin on keto by consuming foods rich in omega-3 fatty acids.

8. Acne. It is expected to see visible improvements in your skin when on a ketogenic diet. It decreases lesions and inflammation in the skin. Also, there is a possible link between consuming high amounts of carbohydrates and increased acne. So, a ketogenic diet helps.

For acne, it would be helpful to limit dairy intake and adopt a stringent regimen for cleaning the skin if you are considering starting a ketogenic diet to improve your skin.

What to Eat and What Not to Eat

When on a ketogenic diet, a few foods are not to be eaten at all, while others are in gray areas. Despite allowing some foods, you still have to ensure that you do not exceed your macronutrient ratios. Simply because a portion of food is allowed does not mean you can keep consuming it as much as you like.

Quality

When fat and protein is concerned, the quality of your food is important. In an ideal manner, you should select meats that are organic, herbivores, and raised with pasture. Eggs should be bought from a local farmer or from hens raised in pastures when possible.

Select grass-derived butter and organic creams, fruits, cheese, and vegetables. Consuming regular foods would not stop you from entering into a ketogenic state, but high-quality foods are more beneficial for your body generally. Ultimately, you are what you eat. Put in your best effort to get the highest quality of food you can obtain or afford.

Fats and oils

The core of your ketogenic diet is made up of fats and oils, so you have to ensure that you are consuming a sizeable portion of them. The ketogenic diet is not just generally fat-free. When on a ketogenic diet, certain fats have greater benefits compared to others, but the ones under some categories may be surprising. While on the ketogenic diet, you should consume sizeable portions of saturated fats in the form of meat, poultry, butter, eggs and coconut, and monounsaturated fats like tuna, mackerel, and salmon. Stay away from highly refined polyunsaturated fats like canola oil, vegetable oil, and soybean oil. Homemade mayonnaise is also a great way to include a dose of fat to each meal.

Proteins

Majority of the fat sources listed previously- meat, poultry, butter, eggs, butter, and fish are also fortified with protein and should be the major source of protein when on a ketogenic diet. Other rich sources of protein that provide a good amount of fat are bacon and sausages.

When consuming protein, ensure that you do not exceed your daily protein requirements because your body converts excess protein to glucose which can stop ketosis.

Fruits and Vegetables

When on a ketogenic diet, most fruits are on the 'not to be consumed' list. Although the sugars in fruits are natural sugars, they still elevate your blood sugar levels if consumed in large quantities and this stops ketosis. There is no tough rule that fruits are not allowed on a ketogenic diet, but the intake has to be restricted. When you consume fruits, select fruits that are rich in fiber and low in carbohydrates like berries, and restrict your portions.

Vegetables are very vital when on a ketogenic diet. They are rich in vitamins and minerals that are required to help you remain healthy, and they also provide a feeling of satiety without adding too many calories. You have to be very picky about the type of vegetables you consume though; since a few are very rich in carbohydrates and are not to be eaten while on a ketogenic diet. Following the general principle, select dark green or leafy vegetables like spinach, broccoli, green beans, cucumber, asparagus, and lettuce. Mushrooms and cauliflower are perfect choices as well. Stay away from starchy vegetables including yam, corn, white potatoes, and sweet potatoes.

Dairy

When on the ketogenic diet, full-fat dairy products are necessary. To meet your fat requirements; Use heavy cream, butter, hard cheese, cottage cheese, cream cheese, and sour cream. Stay away from low-fat dairy products and flavored dairy products like fruity yogurt. Flavored yogurt is rich in sugar in each serving; some types have higher sugar and carbohydrate contents like soda.

Beverages

Concerning beverages, similar to any diet plan, water is the perfect option. Ensure you drink about half of your body weight in ounces. Tea and coffee are also allowed when on the ketogenic diet, but they have to be unsweetened or sweetened with a permitted sweetener like stevia or erythritol. Stay away from soda, sweetened teas, sweetened lemonades, fruit juices, and flavored water.

Grains and sugars

While on the ketogenic diet, stay away from grains and sugars in every form. Examples of these grains are wheat, barley, rice, rye, sorghum and anything produced from them. This implies that no pasta, no bread, no crackers or rice. Sugar and anything containing sugar are also not permitted while on a ketogenic diet. These include corn syrup, maple syrup, white sugar, honey, brown rice syrup, and brown sugar. There are a lot of names for sugar in ingredient lists; it is very important to acquaint yourself with these names so you will be aware when any form of sugar is included on a product.

Chapter 3. Disadvantages of a Ketogenic Diet

Though a lot of adverse effects become evident while adapting to the ketogenic diet, they all stem from the same underlying cause. This section explains what those underlying problems are, the adverse effects related to them and simple techniques to overcome them to enable you to become adapted to the ketogenic diet with as little effort as possible.

The three primary causes

Though, different kinds of symptoms can manifest while on a ketogenic diet, they mostly arise from the same three underlying problems: Hypoglycemia (decreased blood glucose), Hypothalamic-Pituitary-Adrenal axis dysregulation, and Electrolyte and Mineral imbalances. While these three problems seem miles apart, they are in fact connected to each other. Initially, when adapting to the keto diet, your body has been using sugar as an energy source for years, when you unexpectedly change to fats, your body has to construct the cellular mechanisms required to produce and use ketone bodies as a source of energy. The implication of this is that; rather than generating a lot of Ketones initially, for a certain period of time, a lot of people become hypoglycemic. Hypoglycemia disrupts cortisol signaling pathways which in turn causes dysregulation of the HPA axis. Eventually, HPA axis dysregulation results in increased excretion of minerals from the body in the urine.

Together, these three problems cause a variety of adverse effects. As soon as you know this, additional planning can help reduce the probability that these three events will occur.

Hypoglycemia

The foremost underlying problem while adapting to a ketogenic diet is hypoglycemia. This is due to the fact that the body is still inexperienced at burning fat as a source of fuel. During the initial phase of adaptation, people usually feel groggy, tired, intense hunger, depressed, dizzy and irritable.

Though hypoglycemia is not unexpected initially, these side effects should reduce within weeks of starting a ketogenic diet. Watch out for these signs and make plans to support your body during this period.

Keto Flu

This is probably one of the most popular adverse effects of a ketogenic diet. As the name implies, keto flu is when you notice symptoms similar to that seen when you have the flu, and it commences shortly after starting a ketogenic diet. These symptoms include- runny nose, fatigue, nausea, headaches. It is a classic symptom of hypoglycemia that can be managed with basic techniques that will be discussed shortly.

Sugar cravings

A lot of people have noticed that at the earlier stages of a ketogenic diet, they experience severe food cravings. These cravings are for foods rich in sugar and are likely to test your determination.

This is a classic symptom of hypoglycemia too. The brain specifically needs a lot of energy to function properly. When the brain receives a signal that you are hypoglycemic, this sets off a panic response because of a 'primitive instinct' that you are starving to death (although in your conscious state, you are sure you are not). Immediately your brain starts to signal that 'You Need Energy Right Now, or Death is imminent!'; this is when you severely start craving sugar. Fortunately, as soon as you start producing Ketones as a fuel source, you are able to control this panic response.

Dizziness and drowsiness

When you are hypoglycemic and also not completely adapted to a ketogenic diet, in essence, your body's energy stores are depleted. This brief period of adaptation can result in a different adverse effect.

During this period, you will probably feel dizzy and drowsy due to a total lack of energy. Particularly while standing you may feel dizzy, this is as a result of fluctuations in blood pressure and inappropriate cortisol response (which will be discussed soon)

Decreased strength and physical performance

While adapting to a ketogenic diet, you are teaching your body to use a totally different energy source previously unknown to it. The muscles (and also the brain) consists of a lot of mitochondria for production of energy, and they must now learn to use Ketones as a source of energy.

During this period, it is not unexpected for you to experience a drastic reduction in strength and reduced ability to carry out physical activities as one of the temporary adverse effects of a ketogenic diet. Fortunately, once you have fully adapted, you would see significant improvements in these areas than when you were even adapted to sugar.

Hypoglycemia prevention strategies

As already explained, hypoglycemia is responsible for the majority of the adverse effects of a ketogenic diet. These are the top three techniques for controlling these problems:

Eat every 3 hours: Eating every 3 hours in the initial stages of a ketogenic diet helps to keep you feeling 'full' and balances your blood sugar.

Drink beverages rich in minerals: Rather than drinking just water between meals, drink beverages rich in minerals. Examples of these beverages are organic broths or a drink rich in electrolytes.

Eat hydrating foods and food rich in minerals: Eat a lot of hydrating foods rich in minerals and use a lot of salt. I enjoy snacking on cucumbers, celery and particularly Sea Snacks. They are chips containing seaweed that taste amazing and have a lot of fortifying nutrients.

Use Exogenous Ketones: Exogenous Ketones are an incredible way to teach the body to utilize Ketones as a source of energy, instead of having a panic stress response when there is a reduction in blood sugar.

Use Magnesium supplements: If you use these techniques and these symptoms persist, think of including a magnesium supplement in your diet plan. I would recommend taking the L-threonine form on a 1 gram dose between meals three times daily.

HPA Axis Dysregulation

The HPA axis is a combination of three glands (Hypothalamus, Pituitary, Adrenals) that essentially carry out the function of regulating the body's response to stress. When we become hypoglycemic as outlined earlier, the brain goes into a panic mode in response to starvation. The adrenal glands also release cortisol in addition to stimulating sugar cravings. Cortisol directs the release of stores body sugar (glycogen reserves) to provide emergency energy. Due to this response, glycogen reserves are rapidly consumed, there is a recurrence of hypoglycemia, and the cycle goes on. This is when HPA axis dysregulation results in the onset of associated symptoms, at the same time aggravating hypoglycemia related problems.

Disrupted Sleep Patterns

If there is a dysregulation of your HPA axis, it is possible that you will experience a disruption in sleep pattern. This is due to the fact cortisol works against the actions of melatonin. When the HPA axis is dysregulated, cortisol levels are deranged, and this disrupts the proper release time for melatonin.

Cortisol release is triggered by hypoglycemia. Cortisol directs the release of stored glucose in the body, known as glycogen, from the muscle tissue and liver. Cortisol is a stimulating hormone and can interrupt sleep if this occurs at night time. This leads to either insomnia or a reduction in the quality of sleep. Although this cortisol response is beneficial when emergencies arise, it would be better for you to reduce it to as little as possible while adapting to a ketogenic diet and particularly at night.

Heart palpitations

At the initial stages of adapting to a keto diet; most people experience heart palpitations. This can be caused by hypoglycemia, HPA axis dysregulation, and mineral deficiencies.

When the HPA axis is dysregulated, cortisol can become elevated abnormally. If it is constantly elevated, the body becomes cortisol resistant. To match up with the cortisol level in the body, the body starts to produce increased amounts of adrenaline which then results in abnormal heart rhythms.

Also, the deficiencies in minerals which will be explained soon can result in a decrease in blood volume and pressure that can cause the heart to pump at a faster rate or irregularly.

Supporting the HPA Axis

As I have said previously, during the early phase of keto-adaptation, it is possible for the HPA axis to become dysfunctional. At this period, making sure to support the HPA axis in the most suitable way possible would be very beneficial.

Here are my top three techniques that support the HPA axis dysregulation while adapting to keto to decrease the adverse effects of keto.

Techniques to balance blood sugar

Adopt the techniques to control blood sugar as discussed previously. Hypoglycemia is one of the basic triggers of cortisol dysregulation so control this first.

Magnesium supplements: Magnesium is a strong supplement for the HPA axis. Magnesium L-threonate specifically is the only form proven to have the ability to cross the blood-brain barrier which enhances its effects on the pituitary gland and hypothalamus.

Use Adaptogenic Herbs: It is not completely important to use this technique, but using this technique is very advantageous to the HPA axis and help control cortisol levels. Adaptogens can be very beneficial in reducing the adverse effects related to the HPA axis.

Electrolytes and mineral imbalances: Electrolytes and minerals are very important for regulating hydration and also to ensure adequate impulse conduction along the neurons. While adapting to a ketogenic diet, minerals are secreted in excess into the urine as a result of HPA axis dysfunction. This is because, cortisol, together with the HPA axis is responsible for regulating levels of hydration by retaining and secreting minerals. In a way, HPA axis dysfunction can also result in hydration dysregulation. Also, there are other common adverse effects of a keto diet that arise from these deficiencies.

Frequent urination

Increased urination is the most evident sign that your electrolytes and mineral levels are getting depleted. When on a low-carb diet, levels of insulin reduce, and this enhances sodium excretion in the urine. Sodium attracts more water into the urinary system and is then excreted too. This is expected and is one of the vital signs that you are almost fully adapted to the ketogenic diet. Also, your body consumes glycogen reserves in the muscles and liver; additional water is secreted into the urine. Although eliminating this excess water is beneficial in releasing toxins from the body, you have to ensure to take additional fluids, minerals, and electrolytes to prevent other related adverse effects.

Constipation

A very vital sign that indicates inadequate maintenance of electrolytes and mineral balance during keto-adaptation is constipation. The quantity of water contained strongly influences the consistency of your stool and the ability to pass the stool. The quantity of water contained in your stool is thus influenced by your total levels of hydration.

Also, constipation may be an effect of a shift in your natural microflora. The entirety of the bacteria in your digestive system depends on the types of food you consume. When making such an unexpected change in your diet, your microflora changes this temporarily changing the appearance of your stool.

Also know this: Certain foods are likely to promote constipation. Foods such as cheese, nuts, and eggs may contribute to constipation. Restrict your intake of these foods at the initial stages of adapting to keto and notice if that changes anything. Your stool has to pass without straining.

Diarrhea

A few times people will experience diarrhea at the initial stage of a ketogenic diet. Though constipation is generally more common, diarrhea may also arise as a result of the shift in microflora that happens when you change your diet.

Taking a bulking and binding laxative like psyllium, citrus pectin or my preferred one-way activated charcoal would be very beneficial. I advise you to use 2 to 3 grams of activated charcoal every 3 hours until the diarrhea stops.

Also know this: For some people, diarrhea is caused by reduced stomach acid or a slow functioning gallbladder. Another probability is that you have a minor food sensitivity to a food item in a new diet like nuts, cheese, and eggs.

Additionally, if you are supplementing with a large dose of magnesium or Vitamin C, it is advisable to stop this until the diarrhea stops, this could attract more water into the colon. If you add a spoonful of salt to water, it can also act as a laxative. You would try to get your salt in slowly throughout the day by adding a pinch of salt to water and seasoning your food with salt to a suitable taste.

Muscle cramps
Another common side effect of keto-adaptation in the initial phase is muscle cramps. If you notice frequent muscle cramps while becoming adapted to a ketogenic diet, this is probably as a result of mineral deficiencies.

As I have mentioned earlier, minerals are very important for neurons to adequately conduct impulses. A muscle cramp is simply an improperly conducted impulse caused by mineral imbalance and poor hydration.

Ensuring proper hydration and mineral balance
You now know the physiological changes that result in frequent urination, diarrhea, constipation, heart palpitations, and muscle cramps. Luckily, the methods to reduce these adverse effects are very simple. By being a bit more proactive and prepared, the adverse effects of a keto diet will probably be less of a problem.

Top strategies to ensure proper hydration and mineral balance

Hyperhydration: Drink a lot of water, broths rich in minerals and hydrating beverages. You want to make sure any toxins being produced is excreted completely.

Use high-quality salt: Use large amounts of high-quality salts in all your foods. This replenishes sodium and other micronutrients that have been excreted quickly in the initial phases of keto-adaptation. I prefer Himalayan pink or Celtic (gray) sea salt because they are very rich in micronutrients.

Eat mineral rich foods: Add to your intake, foods rich in minerals like leafy greens, cucumber, seaweeds, and celery. As I have said earlier, I enjoy snacking on Sea Snax because they provide a lot of minerals and helps to achieve ketosis.

Use a Magnesium supplement: Except you are experiencing diarrhea, a magnesium supplement is very effective in helping to maintain adequate electrolytes and mineral levels. As you know, magnesium helps keto-adaptation in a number of ways: My general recommendation is using 1 gram in the L-threonate form 3 times every day. If you experience diarrhea, reduce it to once it twice a day till it stops.

Keto Breath

Another side effect that people on a ketogenic diet complain about is keto breath. Though this is not directly as a result of the three major causes previously explained. A lot of people experience keto breath in the initial stages of adapting to keto. When your body begins to produce ketones, you generate them in various forms. Acetone is the form released through the breath and causes the keto breath experienced by some people. Fortunately, acetone is only produced in increased quantity in the early phase of adaptation and reduces very quickly (after 1 to 2 weeks)

Keto Breath Solution

If this is a problem for you, consider brushing your teeth more frequently and using natural breath fresheners all through the day. It is also vital to ensure proper hydration at this period because a dry mouth can aggravate this adverse effect.

Other tested strategies are Oil pulling using coconut oil and using a natural mouthwash when required. I would rather use Oral Essentials mouthwash as it is natural and not as strong as other brands.

Also, you could chew fennel seeds, rosemary, parsley or mint leaves when needed as natural breath fresheners.

Precautions for Certain Situations

For individuals with certain conditions, following a ketogenic diet plan can be therapeutic but strict precautions have to be followed to avoid any severe adverse effects. This is particularly important if you are using medications to manage your condition.

High Blood Pressure: When extremely reducing carb consumption, blood pressure may naturally drop. You might have to discuss this with your doctor before starting at ketogenic diet and make plans to carefully observe your body's response to a diet change.

When you start to experience heart palpitations or feel light-headed, this may be as a result of a drop in blood pressure. It would be beneficial to monitor your blood pressure at this period to evaluate the response of your body to the early phase of adaptation.

People with Diabetes: Because you are consuming less carbs and sugar, you possibly have to reduce your insulin or antidiabetic medications in order to regulate blood sugar.

Also, consult your doctor about this expected change and work with your doctor to fix adequate doses of your medications.

If you experience symptoms like heart palpitations, intense hunger and cravings, lightheadedness and fatigue, this may be a signal that your blood pressure has reduced drastically. Use a blood glucose monitor to evaluate your body's response to the change in diet and ensure that your body is adapting adequately. If important, speak with your physician about medication adjustments.

Exogenous Ketones

Exogenous Ketones is one of the best ways to speed up your body's adaptation to Ketones. They provide an additional form of ketones similar to ketone bodies (Beta-hydroxybutyrate or BHB) produced by our body

Our bodies need time to get adapted to elevated levels of ketones in the body before we can start using them properly and effectively to generate energy for cells. By using an exogenous Ketones supplement, you get your body adapted to ketones quickly and utilizing them as a source of energy before the body builds the metabolic mechanism to successfully generate its own Ketones.

Who Are Exogenous Ketones Beneficial to?

Almost everyone who has been unable to cope with the adverse effects of keto or simply feels uncomfortable on a ketogenic diet would find exogenous ketones very beneficial during the initial phase if adaptation and subsequently.

Also, generating ketones can be very difficult for people who have a weak liver or gallbladder function, have a poor mitochondrial function or are new to the ketogenic diet. In these situations, exogenous Ketones can be very advantageous. Exogenous Ketones are supplements that can be used to provide the body with a source of Ketones that require little to no digestion by the liver and digestive system. This makes them helpful in achieving ketosis and also to provide a quick source of energy and enhance the performance of the body and brain.

Chapter 4. Starting a Ketogenic Diet

Who Should Start a Ketogenic Diet Plan?

If you are struggling with inflammation, try keto.
The keto diet helps you fight inflammation; If you feel sores or aches, you would be happy to know that the ketogenic diet plans help fight inflammation. Sugar stimulates inflammation, and because ketosis burns up fat instead of sugar as a source of energy, a ketogenic diet can prevent insulin spikes caused by an unregulated quantity of sugar that causes an increase in blood sugar and sets off inflammatory reactions in the body.

If you enjoy high-fat foods, try keto.
The ketogenic diet includes lots of fat. If you enjoy high-fat foods such as bacon, red meat, healthy oils, and avocados, you might want to try keto. Eating high-fat foods when you're severely limiting your intake of carbohydrate can alternate it from carb to fat use, promoting greater potential to burn fat in the long term. However, the body doesn't necessarily get any benefit from consumption of bacon, red meat, and avocados aside the use of higher-fat foods as energy,

If you have a body that has high a tendency to store fat, try keto.
Some body types work well with the keto diet. If your body type easily stores carbs as fat, the keto diet is surely a good fit. A big-boned body (endomorph) type fits this class as it is a body

with a higher tendency to store carbs as fat.

If you want to lose weight quickly, try keto.
You can make use of the diet as a "detox." The keto diet can be a short-term solution to quickly lose weight, without worrying about keeping it off for long. If recently, you've gained some weight you wouldn't have otherwise gained maybe you couldn't walk or exercise because you had an injury, or you couldn't get rid of the weight gained from giving birth, you can quickly get back to your regular low weight with the keto diet. You should use it as a "detox" until you have back your normal weight range, a much more sustainable approach to try is including every major food groups.

If you're experiencing continuous heartburn, Try keto.
The keto diet could be of great help. Continuous heartburn, especially the type that comes with a taste of bitterness in the mouth, and or recurring pain in the upper part of the abdomen can be an indication of acid reflux disease. Try the keto diet if you want to help reduce or treat these symptoms.

If you have diabetes, don't try keto.
The risk is not worth it. Keto is not advisable for people with most diabetes' stages, liver disease, or kidney other conditions. Also, the diet may not be a good option for individuals with gestational diabetes, considering the fact that people with that condition have a higher need for protein.

If you're recovering from an eating disorder, don't try keto.
Your body won't get the fat it needs to burn from this diet. If

someone with anorexia is choosing to go on a ketogenic diet, they may get the temptation to do it without taking the adequate amount of fat. This can, however, be dangerous for the body because the ketogenic diet restricts carbohydrates and limits protein. There can be a rapid occurrence of starvation since the fat is also limited, especially in cases where there is no sufficient body fat to burn energy.

If your gallbladder has been removed or if you have had bariatric surgery, don't try keto.

Digestion will be harder for you too. Avoid keto if you have had bariatric surgery because it's harder for your body to absorb fat. You should also avoid this diet if you have had your gallbladder removed, gallbladder disease, or pancreatic deficiency.

Not every patient is a good keto diet candidate, especially patients with chronic conditions like diabetes, high blood pressure, or other conditions which might have been caused by a previous diet.

This diet can cause a huge change in the metabolic and other bodily systems of many people that keeping to the diet may even bring about changes in the effectiveness of their medications.

There is a need for a physician need to be evaluating and monitoring patients when they commence a keto diet because of the extent of dietary restriction. There may be a need for changes in the daily medication dosages they currently take or start an electrolyte supplementation. Speaking with your doctor before you commence is a wise idea.

You'll like to get your water intake level boosted before commencing.

For some patients, there may be a need for sodium supplementation, as long as they're free from blood pressure issues. Some may even need to supplement potassium prescription. As Keto dieters, if you have a continuous hydration issue, you may have to up your carb intake.

Because Keto is not a balanced diet, it is not good as a long-term diet. Any diet devoid of vegetables and fruit will lead to long-term micronutrient deficiencies that can result in other consequences.

As long as a patient is under medical supervision, the keto diet can be useful for short-term fat loss. But it can't be used as maintenance or permanent weight loss solution.

As long as a keto diet is done safely, it is a very effective way for rapid weight loss. In order to solve smaller problems, you don't want to cause bigger ones.

10 Things To Do To Combat Keto Flu Toxins During The 28 Days.

Many of us have had a build up of toxins from years of consuming processed carbs, alcohol, sugars, caffeine, estrogenic foods, unsaturated fatty acids, chemicals, and other foods.

These chemicals and toxins are in our entire system – starting from the cells to the tissues and to our organs.

When you decide to make the necessary changes and to embark in the ketosis journey to become a fat-burner, your body observes the changes and lets you know.

The "keto flu" is the intense detox symptoms you feel in the first phase of ketosis.

It is important to know that the first 7-10 days in the 4-Week Ketogenic Diet will not be so easy, so you want to be adequately prepared to handle the toughness.

You're tough, so to get rid of the keto-flu nastiness, here are some suggestions.

1. Increase your water intake
2. Load yourself with electrolytes
3. Master the art of stress management
4. Have adequate sleep
5. Increase your intake of digestive boosters
6. Drink all three drinks
7. Avoid sedentary living by moving around
8. Be optimistic always
9. Practice patience, be devoted and tenacious

Things to look forward to

There are several other health benefits to be derived from keto dieting (also as you fast intermittently) asides from its fat-burning effects. They include;

- Permanent fat loss which is brought about by calorie deficit
- Reduced cravings
- Trimmed down adipose tissue
- Healthy balance in saturated fatty acid
- Heightened level in growth hormone production (this further increases utilization of fat)
- Trim body mass conservation (fat is lost and is easier to keep off)
- Lessened inflammation
- Lesser risks of developing certain disease conditions such as; cancer, diabetes, cardiovascular diseases
- A cleaner, well-rested and revitalized digestive system
- Increase in lifespan
- Body adaptation associated with 'feeding' on its broken down and ineffective cells, in which these old cells are then replaced, making the body stronger, more vitalized, and more efficient is known to take place. A mechanism

known as autophagy.
- Heightened blood flow to adipose cells causing the removal of these fat cells.
- Reduced insulin
- Increased catecholamines

The list is endless. But by now, you must have gotten the idea. Keto dieting is something you should pursue if you are currently battling with health issues, weight loss but your desired result isn't forthcoming despite every strategy you employed.

If you are expectant, then surely you will see results

'What next?' you might ask

Well, let's take a trip into your future, shall we? In three weeks you'll look better, feel better, and have a great outlook on life and on your eating habit.

Must you keep going?

Yes and no.

Although I believe that keto dieting is a great strategy to adopt when it comes to getting healthy, losing weight and living a remarkably sustainable lifestyle, you still need to 'mix things up.'

I can't speak for anyone else, but I personally get bored eating the same thing and using identical recipes daily. I like to switch things up every once in a while.

This is why I suggest being creative about your ketogenic lifestyle

This is why I recommend switching up your ketogenic lifestyle, with a sustainable metabolism focused approach to eating.

Alternating between keto diet and metabolism approach every three weeks keeps you in high spirit.

In this book, your mind will be prepared by a detailed and direct planner for metabolism boosters which will help you get rid of excess body weight using the keto diet. In the next 3 weeks, you will be able to get rid of swelling, pain, and redness (which are signs of inflammation), boost your metabolism and as such ensuring that you are burning more calorie than you are taking in, balancing your meals, shedding more weight than ever in 21 days.

Are you trying to fight weight gain, and keep it off for good? The main idea of fasting for weight loss is going to be discussed, and then the proper diet, foods, and calories will be discussed later.

Metabolic-detoxifying and kick start keto

Though the whole idea of ketosis as a diet is to make you lose weight. Apparently, your metabolism still plays a major role in making this diet work. If you are told otherwise, please run as fast as your legs can carry you, because you will be damaging your metabolism more.

The very important component of this 3-week ketogenic diet will be detoxing your system, this is done to help clear your metabolic slate apparently, and this will make room for a quicker weight loss which will help you stay motivated for life.

To restart your metabolism and the weight loss process you need to get rid of all the junk foods and proceed to a diet that consists mostly of a wholesome diet, unprocessed foods and totally eliminating foods that hinder your weight loss progress.

At the first phase which is the first-week people normally lose about 4-9 pounds and begin to feel energetic, healthier and really delightful about their new found lifestyle.

Macro-balancing and keto ready

Apart from the detoxification process, another major way of kick-starting the fat burning metabolism is by balancing the three main macronutrients. Since you are getting into ketosis, it pertinent to have the macronutrients in the correct proportion. Balancing your fats, protein, and carbs in their right proportion in your meal is a great way to stabilize your blood sugar rate, calm your digestive system and also regulate your hormonal system.

There is absolutely no one-way of magic when it comes to food and eating. We are all different and as such our bodies respond differently to some food and its combinations. This book will help to show you how you can balance your meals for a greater fat burning experience. We will be starting with rationing your food ratio for evenly balance.

Ketosis

Now as you are trying to maximize your weight loss on the 4-week ketogenic diet, you need to force your body to mobilize as much fat as it can from the fat cells. As earlier discussed a low carb diet is a trick on the body to think there is no food or energy present. So by eating low carb meals, high fat and maybe medium protein the body is tricked, and glucose for the body's survival is denied. Apparently, by keeping glucose out of the body, the body will immediately start getting its daily needs of energy from the stored fat in the body. So through this method calorie deficit is created and the body needs to mobilize more fat than usual to sustain the body.

Generally speaking, to have a resilient, energetic, lean and motivated you, we need to use these three techniques to enhance your metabolism.

Chapter 5. How to Get Started

Load your house with only keto-friendly foods, as fast as you can get to a nearby grocery store and purchase enough keto-friendly foods to stock your kitchen, storehouse, fridge, and pantry with these foods.

Ensure you get these foods as soon as you start getting rid of processed foods, carb, and sugar-laden foods. The essence is that it will help stir you from making bad choices of food and lead you to snack on bad food again.

This is a very personal and important decision of your life, so you don't need to rush this about this, all you need do is to rewrite your food list, draw up your meal plan before the shopping and read the labels on any food you need to buy.

Note that you can get the keto-friendly list on the 21-day guide. Immediately you are sure that the fat burning foods in your home then you can start what is called the purge. This is doing away with all the carb, starch, and processed foods. Going this route will help you transit effectively from your old way of eating to a new one, and of course, you will get some encouragement which will motivate you to do more,

Note we are looking at you progressing, not being perfect for now.

Tips for going out days

Busy days leave you no time to prepare homemade meals, so eating out comes handy. Well, as we all know eating out is a great way of coming in contact with friends and family and food will always be present. So when on a low carb diet it can really be trick you will because most joint visit might not have food for those on a diet, but then even though it seems difficult but it still possible for those on a keto diet to have what to eat. You just need some tips and tricks. It is still possible to manage the menus to align with your keto needs. In this book, you will be able to acquire the knowledge on how to manage your eating out on keto, the restaurant you need to check in and the different options you have.

Majorly you can start by adopting these two simple rules

Rule 1. Do away with high carb foods; I don't think anyone on keto needs to be told this. Carbs must be avoided in restaurants though it might be difficult to resist you just have to try. High carb food that must be avoided are

1. Noodles which includes soda and whole grain noodles
2. Rice and it likes which includes barley, millet, and couscous
3. Tortillas and chips is a no-no. Try making guacamole with celery or even salad
4. French fries are a big no, it's too high in starch, and it has to go
5. Bread and pastry is a no-no so don't eat it
6. Sweet sauces are not for you but you can go for cream-based sauces and gravy
7. Side dishes with root vegetables are also high in sugar and starches so avoid them example onions, sweet potatoes, and carrots.

8. Some deserts too unless the restaurant serves diabetic friendly desserts which are equally low in carbs.

Rule 2. You can order meals of protein and fat rich ones that are listed on the menu. Examples of these foods are:
1. Meats: This will be just fine provided it isn't breaded. These include chicken breasts, steaks, and pork.
2. Seafood: These are great for keto dieters, and they are also an awesome source of omega 3 fatty acids. They include shrimps, mussels, fish, crab, squid, etc.
3. Vegetables: You need to take a look at our 15 low carb vegetables to eat while on keto, go make an order if you like any on the list but if none pleases you then go for a salad without the dressing.
4. Eggs: You can have varieties of this though without the toast you can have scrambled, poached or eggs benedict.
5. Charcuterie plate: This is good as an appetizer. For example, cheese and cured meat.

So generally, just avoid grain-based and starchy foods and go mostly for animal, proteins and low-carb vegetables. It has always been difficult when trying to navigate the menu in restaurants when on keto eating but you will be happier for it when you know how to manage your menu.

How to place your order

Even going by the above-given rules, you might still find out that most restaurants don't offer various keto-friendly meals, but to make your hunting experience shorter and convenience. Request for the following meals
1. Ask for entrée meals, then ask for additional vegetables by the side or better still go for a salad than asking for the normal rice, potatoes, and bread

2. Alternatively, you can make do with entrees without any side dish then order for cream, gravy, and blue cheese dressing
3. If you're going for burgers and maybe sandwiches, then go for the lettuce wrap, not the bun.
4. Other healthy options to order for are, butter, olive oil, and vinegar, these are all keto approved
5. Before eating or requesting for sauces find out first if it was prepared with cream or starch.

What restaurants are good

Whether you're visiting fast food joint, ethnic or premium restaurants, they're still countless restaurants that you can order keto meals from but the ones listed below are places you can easily order your meals from These include

Steakhouse and BBQ: If you need chicken, duck, fish, and seafood you can get to some steakhouses to order for them. Steakhouses sell them apart from steaks, and their menus are always very easy to manage. If you're on keto, you can ask for a steak with cream sauce and maybe with some broccoli on the side, this is a very healthy option. Your best bet is just to move over when you're confronted with fries and placed for salad instead.

Mediterranean: these restaurants are keto-friendly; they do have alternatives like fish with fresh seasonal vegetables or tomato and maybe with mozzarella salad with some olive oil. You should know that Mediterranean food is among the healthiest food on earth because of its high omega 3 fatty acid content, from seafood monounsaturated fats.

Chinese: Another great food you can go for is Chinese foods like stir-fried beef, roasted duck, egg foo young and pork belly. Chinese has so many food options so you will always find something that suits your diet on their menu. You can check out the six keto friendly Chinese meals for more food ideas.

Seafood and Japanese: Normally, Japanese restaurants served mostly different kinds of seafood-based meals, and others are still doing so, so you can think of placing orders for staples like the grilled fish, grilled chicken, or sashimi. Don't go for sushi since it contains rice; this meal isn't healthy for a keto diet. So even if it isn't a Japanese restaurant, you can check out other keto friendly places for your meals.

Buffet: This is a food system that allows you to choose what will be pleasant for your keto palate and good enough some buffets cater for keto dieters, they have meals like grilled fish, steamed vegetables, salads, roasted turkey and even gravy, so you can go for them but avoid salad dressings, sprouted vegetables and tuna because they have mold, bacteria, and toxins in them

It's on record that there should be a great concern when it comes to food served in a restaurant keep away from food people are not willing to eat, it might have been there for a very long time.

Sample keto restaurant meals

The sample below will give you a better view of how your typical meals should look like on a keto diet. Take a look at these different meals you can request for

Breakfast: most restaurants have bacon and eggs on their menu you can order for them; if not you can choose omelet or scrambled eggs. It's on record that eggs are a great source of protein so you can have them, but anytime you get tired of them then try out a Mexican breakfast bowl.

Lunch: You can go for a very simple dishes like a Caesar salad, chicken, smoked salmon or an avocado salad. Be sure to make your lunch to be energy dense as you can. Studies have shown that it better to consume more energy giving food at lunch than for dinner.

Dinner: request for a meat-based entrée with some vegetables and maybe with sauces to liven up the meals. You can alternatively go for fish, shrimp, oysters, mussels, etc. they are all great options.

If you feel a slight hunger in between breakfast and lunch you can go for some healthy snack or brunch like pork rinds, bacon wrapped asparagus, guacamole, and deviled eggs. These are all great alternatives.

What you need to watch out for

You need to pay attention to the food you order for, because hidden carbs are everywhere, sometimes if in doubt you can ask the waiter. When ordering for sauce, dips, and spreads you really need to pay attention to them. It is just that some ingredients are thickened with flour and starch while some are sweetened with sugar and honey which isn't good for the body. But then again, they're good ones that contain fat and protein only. Keto friendly ingredients are hollandaise, guacamole, apple cider, cream, vinegar, hot sauce, mustard, mayonnaise but the bad ones to avoid are ketchup, sriracha, teriyaki, balsamic, beverages, BBQ sauce, buffalo sauce.

Some drinks like alcoholic beverages can be taken too but in moderation. They include sparkling water, spirits, dry wines, and light bear but try and keep away from the following:

Dessert wines: Some of these have very high sugar content, so it better to play safe and take only dry wines.

Liqueur: These are never keto friendly, so avoid them, they contain too much sweetener and, some are flavored with fruits.

Dark beer: Limit stout and lager, almost all the dark ones contain a higher rate of carbs than others.

Cocktails: Limit on this as well. It pretty hard to find a low carb version.

Preparing ahead

If you want to stay ahead and progress better in your keto journey then always prepare for eating out. It's on record that people are always tempted when it comes to food out there especially when we are hungry, so not to succumb to pressure when hunger hits, it's good to do the following:

Have a snack at home

There will always be a temptation to snack with your friends, family or co-workers when dining out or in a social gathering. So not to spoil your keto journey you can make your healthy homemade snacks and take them along with you to the gathering, this will help curb your desire to snack on the snack that will be shared in the gatherings.

Search about the restaurant online

Search for keto friendly restaurants that are near you maybe on Yelp or TripAdvisor. If possible check out their menu to ascertain that they will have what you really need

Research keto food beforehand

If you're new to a keto diet, you might find it difficult making orders. To succeed with this diet, you must first know your keto food well so as to order appropriately. If you are very new to this, you can check the ketocademy course to learn everything you will really need to know about keto.

But if you ask me I will suggest you make your meals at home if you're going the keto way, the essence is that you will really know how much of macro you're consuming, again, you will ascertain that you're eating nutrient-dense foods and you are having total control over your meals.

Nonetheless, from, time to time indulgences either in a Restaurant or social gathering won't hurt your keto progress, if you enjoy eating out sometimes you can still go ahead. But try and go for offers of meats, fish, seafood and then eggs, ordering for vegetables, salads, wine, coffee, and cheese wouldn't hurt but be cautious all the same.

Try and following the tips suggested here, make sure you plan your social gathering meals ahead and don't forget with the right information and knowledge at your fingertips any restaurant can be the right place for your meals. The best bet is to choose and order wisely.

Chapter 6. 28-Day Diet Plan

Week 1

Staying pretty simple at first is our foremost goal here. Simplicity is fundamental for an individual that is just beginning a diet that is low in carbohydrates to me. As an individual, you don't want it to be a challenging transition (kitchen-wise I mean). This is because it will be difficult to just get rid of cravings you have.

Something else we will take into consideration is Leftovers. In addition to the fact that it is less challenging for you, why subject yourself to the hassle of cooking the same food more than one time? Something I do leftover style for is breakfast, where I don't need to worry about it in the morning, and I surely don't need to stress about it. I get some food out of the fridge, which has been pre-made for me and head out of the house. It doesn't get less demanding than that, right?

"Keto flu" where headaches, brain fogginess, exhaustion, and such things can really rile your body up is known as the initial signs of ketosis. Ensure that you're drinking a great amount of water and eating a great deal of salt too. This ketogenic diet is actually a natural diuretic, and you will be urinating much more than you normally do. Take cognizance of the fact that what you're urinating out is electrolytes, and you can figure out that you'll be having a pounding headache in little or no time. It is highly imperative to ensure that your salt intake and water intake is kept high enough, enabling your body to re-hydrate and re-supply you with electrolytes. If doing this does not get rid of the headache totally, it will help with the headaches.

Drink water that contains a sprinkling of salt if you have to. Just continue to drink water (4 liters per day is what I recommend), and continue to eat salt. Trust me, it is going to help. In the event that you have worries about high blood pressure and salt, do not be! The intake of sodium and blood pressure are not really as correlated as we once believed going by recent examinations.

Breakfast.

You want to have something that's quick, not difficult, tasty, and certainly – gives you leftovers for breakfast. I propose beginning day one on a weekend. You can prepare something that is going to last you for the whole week this way. The first week is mainly about simplicity. No one wants to have to make breakfast before going to work, and we will not be doing that either!

Lunch.

Here, we will also be keeping it simple. More often than not, it's going to be salad and meat, slathered in high-fat dressings and then calling it a day. We would prefer not to get excessively rowdy here. Leftover meat from the previous nights or easily accessible canned chicken/fish can be used. Endeavor to read the labels and purchase the one that uses the least (or none at all) additives if you utilize canned meats!

Dinner.

Dinner is going to be a combination of leafy greens (regularly broccoli and spinach) in addition to some meat. Once more, we'll be going moderate on the protein and high on the fat.

P.S. For the initial 14 days, no dessert.

Shopping List

Meat

- Chicken Thighs
- Chicken Sausage
- Canned Chicken
- Bacon

Eggs

- Shrimp
- Stew Meat
- Ground Beef

Fats

- Coconut Oil
- Unsalted Butter (Grass fed)
- Bottle Olive Oil
- Heavy Cream
- Pecans
- Half n' Half

Sauces

- Chicken Stock
- Beef Broth
- Coconut Milk
- Ranch Dressing (Full Fat)
- Dijon Mustard
- Soy Sauce
- Red Wine

Tomato Paste

- Worcestershire
- Tomato Sauce

Cheese

- Queso Fresco Cheese
- Parmesan Cheese
- Cheddar Cheese (Full Fat)

Vegetables

- 6 Lemons
- 3 Onions
- 1 Green Pepper
- Green Beans
- Cauliflower

- Broccoli
- Spinach (lots of this)
- Parsley
- Orange

Spices

- Cayenne Pepper
- Black Pepper
- Bay Leaf
- Allspice
- Chives
- Cardamom
- Chili Powder

Coconut Flour

- Coriander
- Yellow Curry Powder
- Minced Garlic
- Ginger
- Red Pepper Flakes
- Cumin
- Paprika
- Oregano

- Onion Powder
- Salt
- Xanthan Gum

Day One to Seven[1]

Day One

Breakfast. Frittata Muffins (2 Muffins)

One Serving: 27.3g Protein, 32.3g Fats, 2.5g Net Carbs, and 410 Calories

Lunch. Spinach Salad & Canned Chicken

One Serving (3 Tbsp Olive Oil, 1/3 Cup Canned Chicken, & 2 Cups Spinach): 0.5g Net Carbs, 44g Fats, 13.5g Protein and 450 Calories

Dinner. Red Pepper Salad (Add 1 Tablespoon Butter)Inside Out Bacon Burger (1 1/2 Patties) (keep Leftovers in the refrigerator)

One Serving: 4.7g Net Carbs,52.5g Fats,37g Protein and 641 Calories

Totals for the day. 7.7g Net Carbs, 139.8g Fats, 77.8g Protein, and 1601 Calories

Day Two

Breakfast. Cheesy Scrambled Eggs

---

[1] [online] Available at: https://www.coursehero.com/file/p2gk19t/Spinach-Salad-4-Cups-Spinach-4-Tbsp -Olive-Oil-3-Tbsp -Leftover-Meat-624-Calories/ [Accessed 24 Feb. 2019].

One Serving:1.2g Net Carbs, 43g Fats, 19g Protein and 453 Calories

Lunch. Leftover Spinach Salad & Inside Out Bacon Burger (3 Tablespoon Leftover Meat, 4 Tablespoon Olive Oil, & 4 Cups Spinach)

One Serving: 1.2g Net Carbs, 63.9g Fats, and 10.8g Protein and 624 Calories

Dinner. Orange Beef Stew (consume 80% of Whole Stew) & Cinnamon

One Serving: 4.1g Net Carb, 35.6g Fats, 42.8g Protein and 519 Calories

Totals for the day. 6.5g Net Carbs,142.5g Fats,72.6g Protein and 1596 Calories

Day Three

Breakfast. Frittata Muffins (2 Muffins)

One Serving: 2.5g Net Carbs, 32.3g Fats, 27.3g Protein and 410 Calories

Lunch. Simple Spinach Salad (No Meat) (4 Tablespoon Olive Oil and 4 Cups Spinach)

One Serving: 1g Net Carbs,57g Fats, and 537 Calories

Dinner. Chicken Thigh(Curry Rubbed) (1 Chicken Thigh), Fried Queso Fresco (1/4 Pound Fried Queso)

One Serving: 0.6g Net Carbs,44.7g Fats, 40.3g Protein and 657 Calories

Totals for the day. 4.1g Net Carbs, 134g Fats, 72.6g Protein and 1604 Calories

Day four

Breakfast. Cheesy Scrambled Eggs

One Serving: 1.2g Net Carbs, 43g Fats, 19g Protein and 453 Calories

Lunch. Leftover Spinach Salad & Curry Rub Chicken (1/3 Cup Leftover Chicken, 4 Tbsp Olive Oil & 4 Cups Spinach)

One Serving: 1g Net Carbs, 58g Fats, 15g Protein and 586 Calories

Dinner. Bacon Sausage Stir Fry & Chicken (consume 1/3 of Total Recipe) (Freeze 2 Portions as Leftovers) (Add 1/4 Cup Shredded Cheddar Cheese)

One Serving: 8.3g Net Carbs, 38.3g Fats, 42.7g Protein and 541 Calories

Totals for the day. 10.5g Net Carbs, 140g Fats, 76.7g Protein and 1580 Calories

Day five

Breakfast. Frittata Muffins (2 Muffins)

One Serving: 2.5g Net Carbs, 32.3g Fats, 27.3g Protein and 410 Calories

Lunch. Leftover Spinach Salad & Chicken Sausage (2 Tablespoon Olive Oil, Leftover Sausage Stir Fry (1/2 Portion), & 4 Cups Spinach)

One Serving: 4.7g Net Carbs, 70.2g Fats, 20.8g Protein and 742 Calories

Dinner. Cauliflower Curry & Shrimp (consume 1/6 of Total Recipe) (Freeze the remaining 5 Portions as leftovers) (Add 1 Tablespoon Coconut Oil)

One Serving: 5.6g Net Carbs, 33.5g Fats, 27.4g Protein and 451 Calories

Totals for the day. 12.8g Net Carbs, 136g Fats, 75.5g Protein and 1602 Calories

Day six

Breakfast. Cheesy Scrambled Eggs

One Serving: 1.2g Net Carbs, 43g Fats, 19g Protein and 453 Calories

Lunch. Spinach Salad & Canned Chicken (1/3 Cup Leftover Chicken, 2 Tablespoon Olive Oil & 2 Cups Spinach)

One Serving: 0.5g Net Carbs, 31g Fats, 15.5g Protein and 351 Calories,

Dinner. Chorizo & Cheddar Meatballs (consume 5 Meatballs) (Freeze the Leftovers), Roasted Pecan Green Beans (consume 1/6 of Total Recipe) (preserve 5 Portions as Leftovers)

One Serving: 7.1g Net Carbs, 63g Fats, 40.2g, Protein, and 798 Calories

Totals for the day. 8.8g Net Carbs, 137g Fats, 74.7g Protein and 1602 Calories

Day seven

Breakfast. Cheesy Scrambled Eggs (Add 1 Tablespoon Extra Butter)

One Serving: 1.2g Net Carbs,54g Fats, 19g Protein and 553 Calories

Lunch. Spinach Salad & Cream Cheese (1 Oz. Cream Cheese, 3 Tablespoon Olive Oil & 4 Cups Spinach)

One Serving: 2g Net Carbs,51g Fats, 5g Protein and 496 Calories

Dinner. Not Your Caveman's Chili (consume 1/4 of Total Recipe) (Refrigerate 3 Portions as Leftovers), Bacon Infused Sugar Snap Peas (Consume 1/3 of Total Recipe) (preserve 2 Portions as Leftovers)

One Serving: 9.6g Net Carbs, 31.1g Fats, 53.1g Protein and 545 Calories

Totals of the day. 12.8g Net Carbs, 136.1g Fats, 77.1g Protein and 1594 Calories

Week 2

Week 1 is over, amazing. I want to believe you're still doing admirably well on the diet and have found out that it is pretty easy breezy to keep on track with everything!

We will be keeping it simple for breakfast again this week. We will be introducing bulletproof coffee. This is a blend of butter, coconut oil, and heavy cream inside your coffee. If this mixture repulses you - and I know a few of you are saying "WHAT?" - Simply put some trust in me!

This mixture is not as weird as it sounds. After all, butter is made out of cream. So mixing the oil, butter, and cream together simply adds a richness that is decadent to your coffee, and I am very certain you'll truly like it!

Breakfast.

We will be switching it up a bit for breakfast. This is where we introduce bulletproof coffee. At this point, don't misunderstand me – I know a few of you will not like it. Try it with tea on the off chance that you are not a coffee fan. Try making a blending of the ingredients independently and eating it like that if you are not a fan of the taste (which is not very common).

So, why bulletproof coffee?

Loss of fat. Simple and Plain, in both animals and human beings, medium-chain triglycerides (MCT) intake has been shown to cause greater losses in adipose tissue (fat tissue).

Fats! Do I even have to explain this one? Fat consumption has been demonstrated to cause greater energy measures, energy usage that is more efficient, and weight reduction that is more effective. It is also the foremost part of this diet.

More Amounts of Energy. The quick oxidation rate in MCFAs (Medium Chain Fatty Acids) causes an increase in energy expenditure as shown by studies. MCFAs are primarily converted into ketones (Our best companions), are absorbed differently in the body when compared to regular oils, and provide us with more overall energy.

If you're not the biggest fan of the taste, do not hesitate to add sweetener and spices to this. Cinnamon, stevia or vanilla extract. Whatever you'd want to make it taste extraordinary. Just so you don't get bored, you can even switch up the taste every single day!

I advise taking 1-2 hours or so to drink bulletproof coffee down if this is your first time drinking it. Usually, when individuals are greatly exposed to coconut oil which they're not used to, they may have to visit the bathroom regularly because of this. Before drinking it within a time span of 20 minutes, ensure you build a tolerance to coconut oil.

Lunch.

We will still keep it simple here. Into each lunch we make, we can include more meat from the previous night of cooking. Vegetables that are green and high-fat dressings (or vinaigrettes) are vital. It is highly imperative to ensure that the fats balance out with the amounts of protein.

Dinner.

Once again, Dinner is going to be pretty simplistic. The center of our life are Meats, vegetables, high-fat dressings. Since we are getting friskier, probably even a slathering of butter on our vegetables. In the initial two weeks, do not overthink things; note that simple is success.

P.S. No dessert for this week as well, we'll be delving into that next week.

Shopping List

Meat

- Chorizo Sausage
- Chicken Breast

Sauces/Liquids

- Hot Sauce
- Apple Cider Vinegar
- Yellow Mustard
- Coffee

Crunch

- Pork Rinds
- Pecans
- Almonds

Cheese

- Mozzarella Cheese

- Cream Cheese
- Blue Cheese Crumbles

Vegetables

- Sugar Snap Peas
- Green Beans
- Mushrooms
- Lemons
- Spring Onion

Spices

- Mrs. Dash Table Blend
- Baking Powder
- Tone's Southwest Chipotle Seasoning
- Baking Soda

Specialty Items

- Milled Flax Seed
- Almond Flour

Day Eight to Fourteen[2]

Day Eight

Breakfast. Bulletproof Coffee

One Serving: 1g Net Carbs, 30g Fats, 0g Protein and 273 Calories

Lunch. Spinach Salad & Canned Chicken (2 Tablespoon Olive Oil, 2/3 Cup Leftover or Canned Chicken & 4 Cups Spinach)

One Serving: 1g Net Carbs, 32g Fats, 27g Protein and 416 Calories

Dinner. Leftover Chorizo Meatballs (Consume 6 Meatballs), Roasted Pecan Green Beans (consume 1 Portion) (Use Leftovers)

One Serving: 7.9g Net Carbs, 72.2g Fats, 47.5g Protein and 921 Calories

Totals for the Day. 9.9g Net Carbs, 134.2g Fats, 74.5g Protein and 1610 Calories

Day Nine

Breakfast. Bulletproof Coffee

One Serving: 1g Net Carbs, 30g Fats, and 0g Protein and 273 Calories

Lunch. Bacon Mug Cake, Chive & Cheddar

---

[2] [online] Available at: https://www.coursehero.com/file/p2gk19t/Spinach-Salad-4-Cups-Spinach-4-Tbsp-Olive-Oil-3-Tbsp-Leftover-Meat-624-Calories/ [Accessed 24 Feb. 2019].

One Serving: 5g Net Carbs, 55g Fats, 24g Protein and 573 Calories

Dinner. Cauliflower Curry and Leftover Shrimp (Double Serving) (Use Leftovers) (Add 1 Tbsp Extra Butter)

One Serving: 11.2g Net Carbs, 39g Fats, 54.8g Protein and 661 Calories

Totals of the Day. 17.2g Net Carbs, 135g Fats, 78.8g Protein and 1607 Calories

Day Ten

Breakfast. Bulletproof Coffee

One Serving: 1g Net Carbs, 30g Fats, 0g Protein and 4.7g Net Carbs

Lunch. Taco Tartlets (Keto Friendly) (consume 2 Tartlets) (Store / Freeze Leftovers)

One Serving: 5.47g Net Carbs, 38.8g Fats, 26.2g Protein and 481 Calories

Dinner. Curry Rub Chicken Thighs (consume two Total Chicken Thighs) (Make one Extra Chicken Thigh for Tomorrow's Lunch), Red Pepper Spinach Salad

One Serving: 4.8g Net Carbs, 57.8g Fats, 50.3g Protein and 763 Calories,

Totals for the day. 11.2g Net Carbs, 133.5g Fats, 76.4g Protein and 1577 Calories

Day Eleven

Breakfast. Bulletproof Coffee

One Serving: 1g Net Carbs, 30g Fats, 0g Protein and 273 Calories

Lunch. Spinach Salad & Leftover Chicken Thigh (2 Tablespoon Olive Oil 1 Leftover Chicken Thigh & 4 Cups Spinach)

One Serving: 1.6g Net Carbs 47.9g Fats, 24.1g Protein and 553 Calories

Dinner. Buffalo Chicken Strips (Consume 1/3 of Total Recipe) (keep 2 Strips in the refrigerator, Freeze Leftovers), Bacon Infused Sugar Snap Peas (Consume 1 Portion)

One Serving: 9.1g Net Carbs, 58.7g Fats, 42.3g Protein and 750 Calories,

Totals for the Day. 11.8g Net Carbs, 136.5g Fats, 66.5g Protein and 1577 Calories

Day Twelve

Breakfast. Bulletproof Coffee

One Serving: 1g Net Carbs, 30g Fats, 0g Protein 273 Calories

Lunch. Chicken Strip Sliders (Store Almond Buns)

One Serving: 4.3g Net Carbs, 51g Fats, and 34.8g Protein and 625 Calories

Dinner. Omnivore Burger with Almonds and Creamed Spinach (Consume 1/2 Total Recipe) (Keep Leftovers in the refrigerator), Almond Flax Slider Bun (Use Leftovers) (Add One Tablespoon Butter to Almond Flax Slider Bun)

One Serving: 5.3g Net Carbs, 59.9g Fats, 49.1g Protein and 773 Calories

Totals for the Day. 10.6g Net Carbs, 140.8g Fats, 83.9g Protein and 1671 Calories

Day Thirteen

Breakfast. Bulletproof Coffee

One Serving: 1g Net Carbs, 30g Fats, 0g Protein and 273 Calories

Lunch. Spinach Salad & Omnivore Burger (2 Tablespoon Olive Oil 1/2 Leftover Omnivore Burger, & 4 Cups Spinach)

One Serving: 2.4g Net Carbs, 42g Fats, 25.9g Protein 510 Calories

Dinner. Bacon Mozzarella Meatballs (Eat 5 Meatballs) (Freeze Leftovers) Roasted Pecan Green Beans (Consume 1 Portion) (Use Leftovers)

One Serving: 6.7g Net Carbs, 63.8g Fats, 54g Protein and 821 Calories

Totals for the Day. 10.2g Net Carbs, 135.8g Fats, 79.9g Protein and 1605 Calories

Day Fourteen

Breakfast. Bulletproof Coffee

One Serving: 1g Net Carbs, 30g Fats, 0g Protein and 273 Calories,

Lunch. Spinach Salad & Leftover Mozzarella Meatballs (2 Tablespoon Butter (No Olive Oil) 4 Leftover Meatballs, &4 Cups Spinach)

One Serving: 3g Net Carbs, 51.2g Fats, 35.2g Protein and 641 Calories

Dinner. Bacon Sausage & Chicken Stir Fry (Consume 1 Portion) (Use Leftovers), (1 Tablespoon Butter & Add 1/4 Cup Shredded Cheddar Cheese)

One Serving: 8.3g Net Carbs, 49.3g Fats, 42.7g Protein and 641 Calories

Totals for the Day. 12.4g Net Carbs, 130.5g Fats, 77.9g Protein and 1555 Calories

Week 3

We will be introducing a slight fast this week. In the morning, we will get full from fats and fast all the way until it is time for dinner. Apart from the fact that this offers a myriad of health advantages, it's also less difficult on our eating schedule (and schedule for cooking). I recommend eating (drinking rather) your breakfast at 7' o'clock in the morning and then having dinner when it is 7 pm. Keeping a time frame of 12 hours between your two meals. Your body will be put into a fasted state due to this.

Human bodies can break down extra fat that's put away for the energy it needs when in a fasting state. Our body already mimics a fasting state when we are in ketosis, being that we have little to zero glucose contained in our bloodstream, so we utilize the fats available in our bodies as an energy source.

Intermittent fasting is utilizing a similar reasoning – rather than utilize the fats we consume to gain energy; we utilize fat that has been stored away. That being stated, you may believe that it's incredible – you can simply fast and lose more weight. You need to consider that later on, to stay out of a starvation mode, you will need extra fat consumption.

A number of benefits have been shown to come from intermittent fasting. Few of the benefits involved are blood lipid levels, long life, and the truly needed mental clarity.

No big deal if you discover that you cannot do a fast. Return to week 1 and experiment as you deem fit. Provided that it fits into your macros, you can consume what you want.

This is the point where things begin to get more fun - less to stress over, more deliciousness to cook!

Breakfast.

Just like we did in the previous week, we're going full on fats with our breakfast. We'll double the measure of bulletproof coffee (or tea) we drink this time, implying that we double the measure of butter, coconut oil, and heavy cream as well. This should come to quite a considerable amount of calories, and should certainly keep us full till dinner time. To ensure you remain hydrated, and remember to keep on drinking water.

Lunch.

Oh no, No lunch! Don't fret – the fats from your breakfast should keep you feeling energized and full till it is time for dinner. People typically begin to hit a wall at first at around 2 pm, so ensure that you have a great amount of water to drink.

Dinner.

Dinner is staying something similar. Meats, fats, and vegetables are nearly always going to be the dinnertime standard. But you don't have to worry – we'll blend in some bready type things!

Also, guess what, this week we get to have dessert! Woo! For participating in the fasting, we'll be making some low carb and incredibly tasty feasts that will serve as a great reward. Sweets, treats, and weight loss – aren't we lucky?

Shopping List

Meat

- Pork Tenderloin
- Skinless Chicken Thigh, Boneless

Cheese

- Halloumi Cheese (Mozzarella can be substituted)

Sauces

- Spicy Brown Mustard
- Liquid Smoke
- Red Wine Vinegar
- Pesto Sauce
- Red Boat Fish Sauce (or Gluten Free Fish Sauce)

Spices

- Vanilla Extract
- Ground Clove
- Dried Sage
- Dried Rosemary
- Nutmeg

Vegetables

- Lemons

Specialty Items

- Liquid Stevia
- Erythritol

Day Fifteen to Twenty-One[3]

Day Fifteen

Breakfast. Bulletproof Coffee (Double Serving)

One Serving: 1.5g Net Carbs, 60g Fats, 0g Protein and 546 Calories

Lunch. Fasting through lunch, you must drink a lot of water!

Dinner. Chicken Pesto Roulade (consume the whole recipe) Fried Queso (1/4 Pound Queso) (Add 4 Cups Spinach)

One Serving: 3.5g Net Carbs, 55.8g Fats, 75.5g Protein and 886 Calories,

Dessert. Vanilla Latte Cookie (Consume 1 Cookie)

One Serving: 1.4g Net Carbs, 17.1g Fats, 3.9g Protein and 167 Calories

Totals for the Day. 6.4g Net Carbs, 132.9g Fats, 79.4g Protein and 1599 Calories

Day Sixteen

Breakfast. Bulletproof Coffee (Double Serving)

One Serving: 1.5g Net Carbs, 60g Fats, 0g Protein and 546 Calories,

Lunch. Fasting through lunch, you must drink lots of water!

---

[3] [online] Available at: https://www.coursehero.com/file/p2gk19t/Spinach-Salad-4-Cups-Spinach-4-Tbsp -Olive-Oil-3-Tbsp -Leftover-Meat-624-Calories/ [Accessed 24 Feb. 2019].

Dinner. Not Your Caveman's Chili (Consume 1 1/3 Portion) (Use Leftovers)

One Serving: 7g Net Carbs, 23.7g Fats, 69g Protein and 531 Calories

Dessert. Vanilla Latte Cookies (Consume 3 Cookies)

One Serving: 4.3g Net Carbs, 51.3g Fats, 11.7g Protein and 501 Calories

Totals for the Day. 12.8g Net Carbs, 135g Fats, 80.7g Protein and 1578 Calories

Day Seventeen

Breakfast. Bulletproof Coffee (Double Serving)

One Serving: 1.5g Net Carbs, 60g Fats, 0g Protein and 546 Calories

Lunch. Fasting through lunch, you must drink lots of water!

Dinner. Simple Keto BBQ Pulled Chicken (Consume 1/4 Recipe) (Freeze Leftovers) Red Pepper Spinach Salad

One Serving: 6.3g Net Carbs, 50g Fats, 62.5g Protein and 756 Calories

Dessert. Vanilla Latte Cookies (Eat 2 Cookies)

One Serving: 2.8g Net Carbs, 34.2g Fats, 7.8g Protein, 334 Calories

Totals for the Day. 10.6g Net Carbs, 144.2g Fats, 70.3g Protein and 1636 Calories

Day Eighteen

Breakfast. Bulletproof Coffee (Double Serving)

One Serving: 1.5g Net Carbs, 60g Fats, 0g Protein and 546 Calories

Lunch. Fasting through lunch, you must drink lots of water!

Dinner. Inside Out Bacon Burger (3 Total Patties) (Make Use of 290g Beef) One Serving: 2.3g Net Carbs, 69g Fats, 58g Protein and 866 Calories

Dessert. Spice Cake(Low Carb) (Consume one Spice Cake)

One Serving: 3.3g Net Carbs, 27g Fats, 7.3g Protein and 283 Calories

Totals for the Day. 7.1g Net Carbs, 156g Fats, 65.3g Protein and 1694 Calories

Day Nineteen

Breakfast. Bulletproof Coffee (Double Serving)

One Serving: 1.5g Net Carbs, 60g Fats, 0g Protein and 546 Calories

Lunch. Fast through lunch, drink lots of water!

Dinner. Cheddar Bacon Explosion (Consume 1/3 of Recipe) (Refrigerate 2 Portions as Leftovers)

One Serving: 4.9g Net Carbs, 63.7g Fats, 54.7g Protein and 720 Calories

Dessert. Spice Cake(Low Carb) (Eat 1 Spice Cake)

One Serving: 3.3g Net Carbs, 27g Fats, 7.3g Protein and 283 Calories

Totals of the Day. 9.7g Net Carbs, 150.7g Fats, 62g Protein and 1549 Calories

Day Twenty

Breakfast. Bulletproof Coffee (Double Serving)

One Serving: 1.5g Net Carbs, 60g Fats, 0g Protein and 546 Calories

Lunch. Fast through lunch, drink lots of water!

Dinner. Pork Tenderloin (Bacon Wrapped) (Consume 80% of Recipe) Fried Queso Fresco (1/3 Pound Fried Queso)

One Serving: 0.2g Net Carbs, 57.3g Fats, 75.2g Protein and 841 Calories

Dessert. Spice Cake(Low Carb) (Eat 1 Spice Cake)

One Serving: 3.3g Net Carbs, 27g Fats, 7.3g Protein and 283 Calories

Totals for the day. 5g Net Carbs, 144.3g Fats, 82.5g Protein and 1670 Calories

Day TwentyOne

Breakfast. Bulletproof Coffee (Double Serving)

One Serving: 1.5g Net Carbs, 60g Fats, 0g Protein and 546 Calories

Lunch. Fast through lunch, drink lots of water!

Dinner. Leftover Bacon Explosion (Consume 1 Portion) (Use Leftovers) (Add 4 Cups Spinach)

One Serving: 5.9g Net Carbs, 63.7g Fats, 57.7g Protein and 748 Calories

Dessert. Spice Cake(Low Carb) (Eat 1 Spice Cake)

One Serving: 3.3g Net Carbs, 27g Fats, 7.3g Protein and 283 Calories

Totals for the day. 10.7g Net Carbs, 150.7g Fats, 65g Protein and 1577 Calories

Week 4

We will be stricter with our fasting this week. We have had seven days of intermittent fasting, and now we will skip breakfast and lunch. Our BEST friend in this situation is water! Remember to get your liquids in you can take coffee, tea, flavored water e.t.c. To ensure that you're not thinking about your stomach, continue to drink. It MAY begin to growl, simply pay no attention to it – with time your body will adjust.

Now, you can go back and follow week 2 once more if you're the type of individual that can't fast. It is not a big deal, although, I recommend putting your best efforts into it because fasting does take some time for the body to get accustomed to it. The health benefits are not only fantastic, but the self-control that you will gain from doing so is really an incredible thing.

By far, this week is my favorite, and this is because it most closely resembles how I eat on a day to day basis. Normally, I set a window of a time frame of 6 hours for me to eat in. I fast from waking up until it is 5 pm. I am open to eating until 11 pm after this. This is the point where the real fun starts. Consuming copious measures of edibles and being full all through the following day.

With dessert and dinner, you get to begin experimenting more. You get the chance to snack as you wish inside your window and best of everything – you get the chance to eat that protein loaded chicken that you've really been missing so much of!

Breakfast.

Yes, we are fasting! Black coffee in case you're a caffeine addict just like I am. In case you do not really like coffee, Tea. Just like coffee also, tea can add incredible health benefits. Some of green tea's incredible benefits are:

Polyphenols – These function as antioxidants in the human body. Epigallocatechin gallate (EGCG) is the most powerful antioxidant in green tea, and it has been shown as effective against fatigue.

Improved Function of the Brain– in addition, Green tea contains an amino acid, L-theanine, not just caffeine. Your GABA activity is increased by L-thiamine; this improves anxiety, dopamine, and alpha waves.

Increased Rate of Metabolism – Green tea has been demonstrated to improve your rate of metabolism. If it is in combination with the caffeine, this could cause up to 15% increased oxidation of fat.

Lunch.

Water, water, and some more water even after. You don't get to have lunch, and you don't get to have breakfast. So ensure that you keep yourself VERY hydrated. Here, it's important that you do a superb job with your hydration. Do not forget – I prescribe 4 liters daily.

Dinner.

A great amount of food with dessert to cover up the bases! As for me, dinner is a fantastic time. I propose breaking your fast using a small snack, then eat to your heart's content after about 30-45 minutes. I usually require two meals to get to my macros, and I really think you will have to do likewise.

Shopping List

Fats

- Sesame Oil

Meat

- Ground Chicken

Sauces

- Reduced Sugar Ketchup
- Chili Garlic Paste
- 1 Can Coors Light

Crunch

- Pumpkin Seeds
- Peanuts (or peanut butter)

Cheese

- Mozzarella Cheese
- Cream Cheese
- Blue Cheese Crumbles

Spices

- Red Food Coloring

- Capers
- Five-Spice

Day Twenty-two to Twenty-eight[4]

Day Twenty-two

Dinner. Keto Style Szechuan Chicken (Consume 1/3 Total Recipe) (Freeze Leftovers as 2 Portions), Roasted Pecan Green Beans (Consume 1 Portion) (Use Leftovers)

One Serving: 8.5g Net Carbs, 55.2g Fats, 66.7g Protein and 697 Calories

Dessert. Almond Lemon Sandwich Cakes (consume 4 Sandwich Cakes), (Add 1 Tbsp Butter)

One Serving: 7.3g Net Carbs, 81g Fats, 11.2g Protein and 819 Calories

Totals for the Day. 15.9g Net Carbs, 136.2g Fats, 77.9g Protein and 1517 Calories

---

[4] [online] Available at: https://www.coursehero.com/file/p2gk19t/Spinach-Salad-4-Cups-Spinach-4-Tbsp -Olive-Oil-3-Tbsp -Leftover-Meat-624-Calories/ [Accessed 24 Feb. 2019].

Day Twenty-three

Breakfast. Fast for breakfast. You can have tea or black coffee without added ingredients. Also, you can drink water – drinking lots of water through breakfast is highly recommended.

Lunch. Fast for lunch. You can have tea or black coffee without added ingredients. Though, avoid going above 3 cups of tea or coffee a day. Also, you can drink water –drinking lots of water through lunch is highly recommended.

Dinner. Cheesy Creamed Spinach (Consume 1/2 of Recipe) (Freeze Leftovers), Leftover Meatballs (Consume 5 Meatballs) (Use Leftovers)

One Serving: 8.5g Net Carbs, 93.1g Fats, 60.6g Protein and 1061 Calories

Dessert. Chai Spice Mug Cake (Add 2 Tablespoon Heavy Cream)

One Serving: 5.2g Net Carbs, 52g Fats, 12g Protein and 539 Calories

Day Totals. 13.7g Net Carbs, 145.1g Fats, 72.6g Protein and 1600 Calories

Day Twenty-four

Breakfast. Fast for breakfast. You can have tea or black coffee without added ingredients. Also, you can drink water – drinking lots of water through breakfast is highly recommended.

Lunch. Fast for lunch. You can have tea or black coffee without added ingredients. Though, avoid going above 3 cups of tea or coffee a day. Also, you can drink water –drinking lots of water through lunch is highly recommended.

Dinner. Vegetable Medley (Consume 1/3 of Recipe) (Leftovers should be Freeze)**,** Curry Rubbed Chicken Thigh (Prepare 3 Chicken Thighs)

One Serving: 9.3g Net Carbs, 83.7g Fats, 63g Protein and 1069 Calories

Dessert. Almond Lemon Sandwich Cakes (Consume 3 Sandwich Cakes)

One Serving: 5.5g Net Carbs, 52.5g Fats, 8.4g Protein and 539 Calories

Totals for the Day. 14.8g Net Carbs, 136.2g Fats, 71.4g Protein and 1609 Calories

Day Twenty-five

Breakfast. Fast for breakfast. You can have tea or black coffee without added ingredients. Also, you can drink water – drinking lots of water through breakfast is highly recommended.

Lunch. Fast for lunch. You can have tea or black coffee without added ingredients. Though, avoid going above 3 cups of tea or coffee a day. Also, you can drink water –drinking lots of water through lunch is highly recommended.

Dinner. Simple Spinach Salad (2 Tablespoon Olive Oil, 2 Cups Spinach), Thai Style Peanut Chicken (Consume 1/2 of Recipe) (Freeze Leftovers)

One Serving: 9.3g Net Carbs, 81.5g Fats, 72g Protein and 1003 Calories

Dessert. Almond Lemon Sandwich Cakes (Eat 3 Sandwich Cakes)

One Serving: 5.5g Net Carbs, 52.5g Fats, 8.4g Protein and 539 Calories

Totals for the day. 14.7g Net Carbs, 134g Fats, 80.4g Protein and 1543 Calories

Day Twenty-Six

Breakfast. Fast for breakfast. You can have tea or black coffee without added ingredients. Also, you can drink water – drinking lots of water through breakfast is highly recommended.

Lunch. Fast for lunch. You can have tea or black coffee without added ingredients. Though, avoid going above 3 cups of tea or coffee a day. Also, you can drink water –drinking lots of water through lunch is highly recommended.

Dinner. Coffee & Wine Beef Stew (Consume 1/4 of Recipe) (Freeze 3 Portions as Leftovers), Spinach Salad (2 Tablespoon Olive Oil, 2 Cups Spinach)

One Serving: 4.5g Net Carbs, 76.3g Fats, 65.3g Protein and 1015 Calories

Dessert. Chai Spice Mug Cake (Add 3 Tbsp Heavy Cream)

One Serving: 589 Calories, 57g Fats, 5.8g Net Carbs, and 12g Protein

Totals for the day. 10.3g Net Carbs, 133.3g Fats, 77.3g Protein and 1605 Calories

Day Twenty-seven

Breakfast. Fast for breakfast. You can have tea or black coffee without added ingredients. Also, you can drink water – drinking lots of water through breakfast is highly recommended.

Lunch. Fast for lunch. You can have tea or black coffee without added ingredients. Though, avoid going above 3 cups of tea or coffee a day. Also, you can drink water –drinking lots of water through lunch is highly recommended.

Dinner. Drunken Five-Spice Beef (Consume 1/2 of Recipe) (Freeze Leftovers)

One Serving: 12g Net Carbs, 70g Fats, 66.5g Protein and 1030 Calories

Dessert. Keto Snickerdoodle Cookies (Eat 4 Cookies)

One Serving: 8g Net Carbs, 49.6g Fats, 13.7g Protein and 528 Calories

Day Totals. 20g Net Carbs, 119.6g Fats, 80.2g Protein and 1558 Calories

Day Twenty-eight

Breakfast. Fast for breakfast. You can have tea or black coffee without added ingredients. Also, you can drink water – drinking lots of water through breakfast is highly recommended.

Lunch. Fast for lunch. You can have tea or black coffee without added ingredients. Though, avoid going above 3 cups of tea or coffee a day. Also, you can drink water –drinking lots of water through lunch is highly recommended.

Dinner. Red Pepper Spinach Salad (Consume 1/2 Recipe) Lemon & Rosemary Roasted Chicken Thighs (Consume the whole recipe)

One Serving: 7.7g Net Carbs, 58.5g Fats, 55g Protein and 797 Calories

Dessert. Keto Snickerdoodle Cookies (6 Cookies)

One Serving: 12g Net Carbs, 74.4g Fats, 20.6g Protein and 792 Calories

Totals for the Day. 19.7g Net Carbs, 132.9g Fats, 75.6g Protein and 1589 Calories

Chapter 7. Ketogenic Diet Recipes

Almond Lemon Cake Sandwiches[5]

Makes a total of 10 cake sandwiches. One cake (with icing) will be 1.8g Net Carbs, 17.5g Fats, 2.8g Protein and 180 Calories.

Ingredients

Almond Lemon Cakes

- 3 Large Eggs
- 1/4 Cup Honeyville Almond Flour
- 1/4 Cup Butter
- 1/4 Cup Coconut Flour
- 1/4 Cup Erythritol
- 1 Tbsp Coconut Milk
- 1/4 tsp Salt
- 1 Tbsp Lemon Juice
- 1/2 tsp Almond Extract
- 1 tsp Cinnamon
- 1/2 tsp Baking Soda
- 1/2 tsp Vanilla Extract

---

[5] Keto Bootstrap. (2019). *Almond Lemon Sandwich Cakes Keto Recipe*. [online] Available at: https://ketobootstrap.com/recipe/almond-lemon-sandwich-cakes [Accessed 25 Feb. 2019].

- 1/4 tsp Liquid Stevia
- 1/2 tsp Apple Cider Vinegar

Sandwich Icing

- 2 Tbsp Heavy Cream
- 1/4 Cup Powdered Erythritol
- 4 Tbsp Butter
- 1 tsp Red Food Coloring
- 4 Oz. Cream Cheese

Directions

1. Preheat your oven to a temperature of 325F.
2. Sift and prepare a mixture of almond flour, coconut flour, cinnamon salt, and baking soda.
3. Make a combination of eggs, erythritol, almond extract, vanilla extract, lemon juice, melted butter, coconut milk, vinegar, stevia, and food coloring.
4. With a hand mixer, mix up the wet ingredients into the ingredients that are dry until it is fluffy.
5. Your batter should be divided between your muffin top pans and baked for about 17- 18 minutes.
6. Take it off the oven and allow it to cool on a cooling rack for about 10 minutes.
7. Slice cakes into equal parts and fry the halves in butter until it becomes crisp.

8. Allow it to cool on the cooling rack once more.

9. Make a mixture of cream cheese, heavy cream, butter, and powdered erythritol until fluffy. Continue to add food coloring until desired color is attained.

10. In between the middle of the cakes, divide icing and prepare a sandwich. Garnish it using lemon zest and pistachios.

Inside Out Bacon Burger[6]

Makes 1 Serving (3 patties). One serving will be 1.8g Net Carbs, 51.8g Fats, 43.5g Protein and 649 Calories.

Ingredients

- 1/4 tsp Worcestershire
- 1/4 tsp Onion Powder
- 1/2 tsp Salt
- 200g Ground Beef
- 2 Tbsp Cheddar Cheese
- 2 Slices Bacon
- 1/2 tsp Minced Garlic
- 1 1/2 tsp Chopped Chives
- 3/4 tsp Soy Sauce
- 1/2 tsp Black Pepper

Directions

1. Cook all your bacon that has been chopped until it becomes crisp in a cast iron skillet. Once you are done with cooking, take it off and place on a paper towel. Drain the grease separately and save it.

---

[6] Burger, L. (2019). *Inside Out Bacon Burger | Ruled Me*. [online] Ruled Me. Available at: https://www.ruled.me/inside-out-bacon-burger/ [Accessed 25 Feb. 2019].

2. Make a combination of ground beef, 2/3 chopped bacon, and what is left of the spices in a large mixing bowl.

3. Mix up the meat and spices well, after this form into 3 patties.

4. Place 2 Tbsp bacon fat inside a cast iron pan then place patties inside it once fat becomes hot.

5. Contingent upon the doneness you desire, cook for about 4-5 minutes on each side.

6. Remove from the pan, allow it to rest for about 3-5 minutes, and serve with cheese, additional bacon, and onion if you so desire.

Bacon & Mozzarella Meatballs

Makes 24 medium meatballs. For one meatball, you're looking at: 0.7g Net Carbs, 9.4g Fats, 10.1g Protein and 128 Calories.

Ingredients

- 4 Slices Bacon
- 1 1/2 lb. Ground Beef
- 3/4 Cup Pesto Sauce
- 1 Cup Mozzarella Cheese
- 1/3 Cup Crushed Pork Rinds
- 1 tsp Pepper
- 2 tsp Minced Garlic
- 2 Large Eggs
- 1/2 tsp Kosher Salt
- 1/2 tsp Onion Powder

Directions

1. Preheat oven to a temperature of 350F.
2. Slice your bacon into pieces that are small in size (nearly into small cubes).
3. To the bacon, add your ground beef, ground pork rinds, cheese, spices, and eggs.
4. Mix everything together well until meatballs can be formed.

5. Roll out your meatballs in circles and put them in a foiled baking tray.

6. Bake in the oven for about 40-45 minutes, or until the bacon has been cooked.

7. For each meatball, spoon out 1/2 Tbsp pesto sauce and serve afterward.

Bacon Infused Sugar Snap Peas

Makes 3 total servings. For each Serving, you're looking at: 4.3g Net Carbs, 13.3g Fats, 1.3g Protein and 147 Calories.

Ingredients

- 3 Tbsp Bacon Fat
- 1/2 tsp Red Pepper Flakes
- 3 Cups Sugar Snap Peas (~200g)
- 2 tsp Garlic
- 1/2 Lemon Juice

Direction

1. Add 3 Tbsp of bacon fat into a pan and bring it to its smoking point.
2. Add your garlic to it and reduce the heat on the pan, allowing the garlic to cook for about 60 to 120 seconds.
3. After that add sugar snap peas and lemon juice to it, allow it to cook for about 1-2 minutes.
4. Take it off and serve. Garnish it using red pepper flakes and lemon zest.

BBQ Pulled Chicken

Makes 4 Total Servings. For each serving, you are looking at: 2.3g Net Carbs, 30g Fats, and 51.5g Protein and 510 Calories.

Ingredients

- 1/3 Cup Salted Butter
- 6 Boneless, Skinless Chicken Thighs
- 1/4 Cup Chicken Stock
- 1/4 Cup Erythritol
- 1/4 Cup Red Wine Vinegar
- 2 Tbsp Spicy Brown Mustard
- 1/4 Cup Organic Tomato Paste
- 1 Tbsp Liquid Smoke
- 1 tsp Cumin
- 2 Tbsp Yellow Mustard
- 1 Tbsp Soy Sauce
- 2 tsp Chili Powder
- 1 tsp Red Boat Fish Sauce
- 1 tsp Cayenne Pepper

Direction

1. With the exception of butter and chicken thighs, mix all other ingredients together.

2. Put frozen (or fresh) chicken thighs inside slow cooker and pour sauce over the thighs.

3. Add butter, switch to low and leave it for about 7-10 hours if you will not be home.

4. Allow it to cook on low for 2 hours. Add your butter, switch to high, and then cook for an extra 3 hours if you will be home.

5. Shred the chicken using two forks once your chicken is cooked. Mix up all the sauce together and allow it to cook on high for 45 minutes in the absence of the top. This will decrease the sauce.

6. Optional: With coarse sea salt sprinkled over the top, serve alongside chili paste with a sprinkle of curry powder added for color.

Buffalo Chicken Strips

Makes 3 total servings (9 total strips.) For One serving, the chicken strips come out to 4.8g Net Carbs, 54g Fats, 41g Protein and 683 Calories.

Ingredients

- 1 tsp Onion Powder
- 1 tsp Garlic Powder
- 3/4 Cup Almond Flour
- 5 Chicken Breasts Pounded to 1/2" Thickness
- 1/4 Cup Olive Oil
- 1/2 Cup Hot Sauce
- 3 Tbsp Blue Cheese Crumbles
- 3 Tbsp Butter
- 1 Tbsp Chili powder
- 1 Tbsp Paprika
- 2 Large Eggs
- 2 tsp Pepper
- 2 tsp Salt

Direction

1. Preheat oven to a temperature of 400F.
2. Make a combination of paprika, chili powder, salt,

pepper, garlic powder, and onion powder inside a ramekin.

3. Pound out the breasts of the chicken to 1/2" thickness, then cut the chicken breasts in half afterward.

4. Sprinkle 1/3 of the spice mix all over the breast of the chicken, after this flip them over and do likewise with 1/3 of the spice mix.

5. Make a combination of almond flour and 1/3 of the spice mix in a bowl.

6. Crack 2 eggs and whisk them inside a separate container.

7. Dip each seasoned chicken piece into the spice mix and then dip into the almond flour. Ensure that each side is well coated.

8. On a cooling rack over a baking sheet that is foiled, lay each piece.

9. Bake the chicken for a period of 15 minutes.

10. Remove the chicken from the oven and then turn your oven to broil. Sprinkle 2 Tbsp of olive oil over the chicken.

11. Broil for a period of 5 minutes. Flip the breasts, then sprinkle with the remaining olive oil, and broil once again for a period of 5 minutes.

12. Make a combination of 1/2 Cup of hot sauce with 3 Tbsp of butter in a saucepan.

13. With hot sauce slathering and blue cheese crumbles as well, serve chicken.

Bulletproof Coffee

Yields One total serving. One serving comes out to 1g Net Carbs, 30g Fats, 0g Protein and 273 Calories.[7]

Ingredients

- 1 Cup Coffee
- 1 Tbsp Heavy Cream
- 1 Tbsp Unsalted Butter
- 1 Tbsp Coconut Oil

Direction

1. Brew one cup worth of coffee inside a big container. A measuring cup is what I utilize.
2. Slice off a Tbsp of butter. Drop the butter inside your coffee and let it ooze.
3. Measure a Tbsp of coconut oil and pour that into your coffee as well.
4. Finally, the 1 Tbsp of heavy cream. An incredible creaminess is added to the coffee by this.
5. With a hand blender, mix everything together very well.

---

[7] Ruled Me. (2019). *Perfect Cup of Ketoproof Coffee | Ruled Me*. [online] Available at: https://www.ruled.me/ketoproof-coffee/ [Accessed 5 Mar. 2019].

Chai Spice Mug Cake

Yields One Serving. For one serving this is 4g Net Carbs, 42g Fats, 12g Protein and 439 Calories.[8]

Ingredients

Base

- 1/2 tsp Baking Powder
- 2 Tbsp Honeyville Almond Flour
- 1 Large Egg
- 2 Tbsp Butter
- 7 Drops Liquid Stevia
- 1 Tbsp NOW Erythritol

Flavor

- 1/4 tsp Cinnamon
- 2 Tbsp Honeyville Almond Flour
- 1/4 tsp Cardamom
- 1/4 tsp Ginger
- 1/4 tsp Vanilla Extract
- 1/4 tsp Clove

---

[8] Cake, C. (2019). *Chai Spice Keto Mug Cake | Ruled Me*. [online] Ruled Me. Available at: https://www.ruled.me/chai-spice-keto-mug-cake/ [Accessed 25 Feb. 2019].

Direction

1. Inside a mug, mix up all room temperature ingredients together.

2. Microwave on high for a period of 70 seconds.

3. Turn the mug upside down and lightly strike it against a plate.

4. This is optional: Top it with whipped cream and a sprinkle of cinnamon.

Bacon Cheddar Explosion

Yields three Total Servings. Per serving, you are looking at: 4.9g Net Carbs, 63.7g Fats, 54.7g Protein and 720 Calories.[9]

Ingredients

- 2 tsp Mrs. Dash Table Seasoning
- 4-5 Cups Raw Spinach
- 30 Slices of Bacon
- 1-2 Tbsp Tones Southwest Chipotle Seasoning
- 2 1/2 Cups Cheddar Cheese

Direction

1. Preheat your oven to a temperature of 375 F convection bake. (A temperature of 400F regular bake)

2. You should weave the bacon. 15 pieces of bacon that are vertical, 12 pieces of bacon that are in horizontal form, and the additional 3 cut into half to fill in the rest, in a horizontal manner.

3. Using your favorite seasoning mix, season your bacon.

4. To the bacon, add your cheese leaving about 1 1/2

---

[9] Explosion, C. (2019). *Cheddar Bacon Explosion | Ruled Me*. [online] Ruled Me. Available at: https://www.ruled.me/cheddar-bacon-explosion/ [Accessed 25 Feb. 2019].

inch gaps between its edges.

5. Add your spinach to it and press it down to compress some. When you roll it up, this will help.

6. Slowly, roll your weave ensuring that it remains tight and a lot does not fall through it. Some cheese may fall out, however, you should not worry about it. If you so desire, add your seasoning to the outside here.

7. Foil one baking sheet and add a great amount of salt to it. This will prevent your oven from smoking and aid in catching excess grease from the bacon.

8. Place your bacon over a cooling rack and place that over your baking sheet.

9. Without opening the door of the oven, bake for a period of 60-70 minutes. When it is finished, your bacon ought to be very crisp on the top.

10. Before attempting to take it away from the cooling rack, allow it to cool for a period of 10-15 minutes. Slice it into pieces, and then serve!

Cheddar Chorizo Meatballs

Makes 24 medium meatballs. Each meatball with sauce will give: 0.8g Net Carbs, 7.8g Fats, 9.9g Protein and 115 Calories[10].

Ingredients

- 1 1/2 lb. Ground Beef
- 1 Cup Cheddar Cheese
- 1 1/2 Chorizo Sausages
- 1 Cup Tomato Sauce
- 2 Large Eggs
- 1/3 Cup Crushed Pork Rinds
- 1 tsp Chili Powder
- 1 tsp Cumin
- 1 tsp Kosher Salt

Direction

1. Preheat oven to a temperature of 350F.
2. To ensure that the sausage will mix well with the ground beef, break it up into small pieces.
3. Add the ground beef, ground pork rinds, eggs, spices, and cheese to the sausage.

---

[10] Meatballs, C. (2019). *Chorizo & Cheddar Cheese Meatballs | Ruled Me*. [online] Ruled Me. Available at: https://www.ruled.me/chorizo-cheddar-cheese-meatballs/ [Accessed 25 Feb. 2019].

4. Thoroughly mix all of them together until meatballs can be formed.

5. Roll out the meatballs into circles and put them in a foiled baking tray.

6. Bake meatballs in the oven for a period of 30-35 minutes, or until they are cooked through.

7. Pour tomato sauce over your meatballs and then serve.

Cheesy Scrambled Eggs

Makes 1 serving. Per serving, it is: 1.2g Net Carbs, 43g Fats, 19g Protein and 453 Calories.

Ingredients

- 250ml Cheddar Cheese
- 3 Large Eggs
- 2 Tbsp Butter
- 1 chopped green onion

Direction

1. On the stove, heat a pan. Put the butter in the pan.
2. Once the butter has finished melting, put 3 scrambled eggs with the chopped onion
3. Allow the eggs to cook slowly, touching them only once or twice all through the entire process.
4. Add cheese to it and thoroughly mix everything together.

Cheesy Spinach

Makes 2 servings. For each serving, it is: 4.8g Net Carbs, 47g Fats, 24g Protein and 446 Calories.

Ingredients

- 3 Tbsp Butter
- 7 Cups Spinach
- 1/2 tsp Mrs. Dash
- 1 1/2 Cup Cheddar Cheese
- 1/2 tsp Pepper
- 1/2 tsp Salt

Direction

1. Heat a pan up on the stove, add the butter to it.
2. Add the spinach and spices once the butter has finished melting. Allow the spinach to start wilting.
3. Add shredded cheese to the top once the spinach is almost totally wilted and allow everything to melt together.
4. Once it has melted, serve.

Chicken Roulade

Yields one servings. For one serving, this is 2.5g Net Carbs, 31g Fats, 53.3g Protein and 478 Calories.

Ingredients

- 38g Halloumi Cheese
- Zest 1/4 Lemon
- 1 Chicken Breast
- 2 1/4 tsp Olive Oil
- 1/2 Tbsp Pesto
- 1/4 tsp Garlic

Direction

1. Pat the chicken breast dry to make it free of any extra moisture. Pound your chicken breast to 1/8".
2. Make a mixture of Pesto and 1 1/4 tsp of olive oil. Spread out the mixture on all of the chicken breasts.
3. To each chicken, add salt, pepper, and lemon zest.
4. Add sliced halloumi cheese to chicken breast.
5. Roll up the chicken breast and tie them up utilizing butcher's string or even toothpicks.
6. Preheat your oven up to a temperature of 450F.

7. In a cast iron pan, heat 1 tsp of Olive Oil to high heat.

8. Sear each of the chicken's side ensuring that it gets nice and brown.

9. Bake for a period of 6-7 minutes until juice runs clear.

Buffalo Chicken Strip Slider

Makes 8 Buns (use only 2 in a serving). For a serving, this is 4.3g Net Carbs, 51g Fats, 34.8g Protein and 625 Calories.

Ingredients

Almond Flour Buns

- 1/2 tsp Apple Cider Vinegar
- 1 tsp Paprika
- 1 tsp Baking Soda
- 2 Large Eggs
- 1/4 Cup Flax Seed
- 3 Tbsp Parmesan Cheese
- 1/3 Cup Almond Flour
- 4 Tbsp Butter
- 1 tsp Southwest Seasoning

Chicken Filling

- 2 Leftover Buffalo Chicken Strips

Direction

1. Preheat oven to a temperature of 350F.
2. In a large mixing bowl, mix all the dry ingredients together.

3. In the microwave, melt the butter and then add eggs, vinegar, stevia and butter to the mixture.

4. Mix everything thoroughly and spread out the mixture between 8 muffin top spaces in a pan.

5. Bake for a period of 15-17 minutes. Allow it to cool for 5 minutes once baked, then cut the buns in half.

6. Assemble the slider together with bun, in addition to buffalo chicken strips.

Bacon, Cheddar & Chive Mug Biscuit

Gives 1 Serving. One serving is 5g Net Carbs, 55g Fats, 24g Protein and 573 Calories.[11]

Ingredients

Base

- 2 Tbsp Butter
- 1 Egg
- 1/2 tsp Baking Powder
- 2 Tbsp Almond Flour

Flavor

- 1 Tbsp Chopped Chive
- 2 Slices Bacon
- 1 Tbsp Almond Flour
- 1 Tbsp Packed Shredded White Cheddar
- 1 Tbsp Packed Shredded Cheddar
- Pinch Salt

---

[11] Bacon, C. (2019). *Bacon, Cheddar and Chive Mug Cake | Ruled Me*. [online] Ruled Me. Available at: https://www.ruled.me/bacon-cheddar-chive-mug-cake/ [Accessed 25 Feb. 2019].

Direction

1. Inside a mug, mix all room temperature ingredients together.

2. Microwave on high for a period of 70 seconds.

3. Turn the cup upside down and strike it lightly against a plate.

4. This is optional: allow it to cool for about 3-4 minutes.

Orange & Cinnamon Beef Stew

Yields one serving with leftovers. One serving is Net Carbs, 44.5g Fats, 1.9g, 53.5g Protein, and 649 Calories.

Ingredients

- 1/4 tsp Rosemary
- 1/4 Medium Onion
- 1 Bay Leaf
- 1/4 Pound Beef
- Zest of 1/4 Orange
- 3/4 Cup Beef Broth
- Juice of 1/4 Orange
- 1 Tbsp Coconut Oil
- 3/4 tsp Minced Garlic
- 3/4 tsp Fresh Thyme
- 1/2 tsp Ground Cinnamon
- 1/2 tsp Fish Sauce
- 1/2 tsp Soy Sauce
- 1/4 tsp Sage

Direction

1. Your vegetables should be diced, cut up your meat into approximate 1" cubes. Also, zest an entire orange.

2. In a cast iron skillet, heat up coconut oil, waiting for it till it reaches the smoke point.

3. In batches, add your seasoned (salt plus pepper) meat to the skillet. Don't overload the skillet. Brown the beef and take it away from the cast iron, after this add extra beef to brown.

4. Once your beef is done browning, take away the last batch and then add your vegetables. Allow these to cook for about 1-2 minutes.

5. In order to deglaze the pan, add your orange juice and after this add every other ingredient with the exception of the rosemary, sage, and thyme.

6. Allow this to cook for a moment, and transfer all ingredients into your crock pot after this.

7. Allow this to cook for a period of 3 hours on high.

8. Open up your crock pot and put in the rest of your spices. Allow this to cook down for a period of 1-2 hours on high.

Coffee & Red Wine Beef Stew

Yields 4 servings. For a serving, this is 4g Net Carbs, 48.3g Fats, 63.8g Protein and 755 Calories. (Freeze Leftovers)[12]

Ingredients

- 2 tsp Garlic
- 3 Cups Coffee
- 2.5 Pounds Stew Meat
- 2 Tbsp Capers
- 1 Cup Beef Stock
- 2/3 Cup Red Wine (Merlot)
- 1 1/2 Cup Mushrooms
- 3 Tbsp Coconut Oil
- 1 Medium Onion

Direction

1. Cube all of the stew meat, after this slice onions and mushrooms thinly.
2. Inside a pan on the stove, bring 3 Tbsp of coconut oil to its smoking point.

---

[12] Schwartz, S. (2019). *Coffee and Wine Beef Stew Recipe | The Nosher.* [online] My Jewish Learning. Available at: https://www.myjewishlearning.com/the-nosher/coffee-and-wine-beef-stew-recipe/ [Accessed 25 Feb. 2019].

3. Using salt and pepper season the beef, after this brown all of it in small batches, ensuring that the pan is not overcrowded.

4. Cook onions, mushrooms, and garlic in the fat that is left in the pan once all meat has been browned. Keep doing this until onions are translucent.

5. Add coffee, red wine, beef stock, and capers to the vegetables and stir up this mixture.

6. Include meat in the mixture, let it boil then decrease the heat to low.

7. Cover it up and cook for a period of 3 hours.

Crispy Curry Rubbed Chicken Thigh

Yields 1 serving. For each serving, this is 1.3g Net Carbs, 39.8g Fats, 42.3g Protein and 555 Calorie.[13]

You'll need to make an extra chicken thigh if you are on week 4

Ingredients

- Pinch Ginger
- Pinch Cardamom
- Pinch Cinnamon
- 1 Tbsp Olive Oil
- 2 Chicken Thighs
- 1/2 tsp Salt
- 1/2 tsp Yellow Curry
- 1/4 tsp Garlic Powder
- 1/4 tsp Paprika
- 1/4 tsp Cumin
- 1/8 tsp Coriander
- 1/8 tsp Cayenne Pepper
- 1/8 tsp Chili Powder
- 1/8 tsp Allspice

---

[13] Myfitnesspal.com. (2019). *Calorie Chart, Nutrition Facts, Calories in Food | MyFitnessPal | MyFitnessPal.com*. [online] Available at: https://www.myfitnesspal.com/food/calories/keto-crispy-curry-rubbed-chicken-thighs-282875976 [Accessed 25 Feb. 2019].

Direction

1. Preheat oven to a temperature of 425F.
2. Inside a bowl, mix all the spices together.
3. Wrap up a baking sheet in foil and on to the foil, lay the thighs of the chicken.
4. Evenly rub olive oil into each of the chicken thighs.
5. On each side of the chicken, rub spice mixture. Coat it generously.
6. Bake for a period of 40-50 minutes.
7. Allow it to cool for a period of 5 minutes before serving.

Drunken Five Spice Beef

Yields 4 Total Servings, each coming out to 6g Net Carbs, 35g Fats, 33.3g Protein and 515 Calories. (Freeze Leftovers)[14]

Ingredients

- 1/2 tsp Onion Powder
- 1 tsp Cayenne Pepper
- 2 tsp Cumin
- 1 1/2 lbs. Ground Beef
- 150g Sliced Mushrooms
- 1 Can Coors Light (Or 1/2 Cup Red Wine)
- 75g Raw Spinach
- 135g Chopped Broccoli
- 2 Tbsp Soy Sauce
- 3 Tbsp Reduced Sugar Ketchup
- 1 Tbsp Five Spice
- 2 tsp Salt
- 2 tsp Garlic
- 2 tsp Minced ginger
- 1 Tbsp Pepper

---

[14] Beef, D. (2019). *Drunken Five Spice Beef*. [online] MealPlannerPro.com. Available at: https://mealplannerpro.com/member-recipes/Drunken-Five-Spice-Beef-905141 [Accessed 25 Feb. 2019].

Direction

1. Chop broccoli florets, ginger, and garlic as well.

2. Heat a cast iron pan to high heat then add ground beef.

3. Brown all of the ground beef, after this, add ginger and garlic into the pan.

4. Mix up everything thoroughly, add broccoli and spices then mix everything up together.

5. Pour a can of Coors Light (or any other low carb beer, or half Cup of Red Wine) inside the pan. Add mushrooms and spinach to the mixture then mix everything up together.

6. Add ketchup, mix, and serve once the spinach has wilted!

Cheesy Frittata Muffins

Yields 8 servings, each having 1.3g Net Carbs, 16.1g Fats, 13.6g Protein and 205 Calories.[15]

Ingredients

- 4 Oz. Bacon (pre-cooked and chopped)
- 1/2 Cup Cheddar Cheese
- 1/2 tsp Pepper
- 1/2 Cup Half n' Half
- 8 Large Eggs
- 2 tsp Dried Parsley
- 1 Tbsp Butter
- 1/4 tsp Salt

Direction

1. Preheat oven to a temperature of 375 degrees
2. In a bowl, mix the eggs together and half n' half inside a bowl until it is nearly scrambled, leaving egg white streaks.
3. Fold in bacon, spices, and cheese. Any other additional ingredients ought to be added now

---

[15] Eat This Much, I. (2019). *Eat This Much, your personal diet assistant.* [online] Eat This Much. Available at: https://www.eatthismuch.com/recipe/nutrition/cheesy-frittata-muffins,364652/ [Accessed 25 Feb. 2019].

4. Grease a muffin tin using butter. This formula makes around 8 frittata muffins.

5. Pour the mixture in the cup, filling each of the cups until it is about ¾ full.

6. Stick them inside the oven for a period of 15-18 minutes, or until the edges turn puffy and golden.

7. Take it away from the oven and allow it to cool for 60 seconds. These freeze well and can be also be heated individually.

Fried Queso Fresco

Makes 5 servings. For each serving, it is 0g Net Carbs, 19.5g Fats, 16g Protein and 243 Calories. (Save Leftovers)[16]

Ingredients

- 1/2 Tbsp Olive Oil
- 1 Tbsp Coconut Oil
- 1 lb. Queso Fresco

Direction

1. Cut up the cheese into cube shapes, or into thin rectangles.
2. Inside a pan, bring 1 Tbsp of coconut oil and 1/2 Tbsp of olive oil to high heat.
3. Add your cheese once the smoke point is hit. Allow it to cook until it is browned on a side and then flip it over and do likewise on the other side.
4. Take it away from the pan and drain grease that is in excess on a paper towel.

---

[16] OneEarthHealth. (2019). *Fried Queso Fresco.* [online] Available at: https://oneearthhealth.com/blogs/keto-recipes/fried-queso-fresco [Accessed 25 Feb. 2019].

Lemon Rosemary Chicken

Yields 1 serving. Per serving, it is 4.2g Net Carbs, 40.5g Fats, 47g Protein and 589 Calories.

Ingredients

- 1/2 tsp Dried Ground Sage
- 3/4 tsp Dried Rosemary
- 3 1/2 Skinless and Boneless Chicken Thigh (Cut 1 thigh in half to get 1/2,)
- 1 1/2 tsp Fresh Thyme
- 1 1/2 tsp Olive Oil
- 1 Lemon
- 1 1/2 tsp Minced Garlic

Direction

1. Inside a mortar, add your garlic and 1 tsp of kosher salt
2. Using a pestle grind the garlic and salt together, making a paste.
3. Add your oil slowly, grinding and mixing up the paste into an aioli.
4. Once the aioli is done, dry off your chicken and place it into a bag with the aioli. Make sure you coat the chicken well.
5. Marinate your chicken for a period of 2-10

hours.

6. Preheat your oven to a temperature of 425F.

7. Slice up 1 lemon thinly and arrange the slices on a baking pan's base.

8. Lay your chicken over the lemons.

9. Take the thyme leaves away from the stem then add your thyme, rosemary, sage, pepper, and what is left of the salt to your chicken.

10. Bake in the oven for about 25-30 minutes, or till the juices run clear.

11. Take the chicken off the pan and pour all of the pan drippings into a saucepan.

12. While stirring thoroughly, bring the sauce to boil.

13. Turn the heat down to medium-low heat while still stirring the sauce. Allow it to decrease.

14. Pour the sauce all over the chicken, enjoy it!

Keto Szechuan Chicken

Makes 3 Total Servings, each yielding 5.2g Net Carbs, 38.3g Fats, 63g Protein and 515 Calories. (Freeze Leftovers)[17]

Ingredients

- 1/2 tsp Minced Ginger
- 1/2 tsp Mrs. Dash Table Blend
- 1 tsp Red Pepper Flakes
- 2 tsp Pepper
- 2 Tbsp Soy Sauce
- 2 Tbsp Chili Garlic Paste
- 1/2 Cup Chicken Stock
- 6 Cups Spinach
- 1 1/2 lbs. Ground Chicken
- 3 Tbsp Coconut Oil
- 4 Tbsp Organic Tomato Paste
- 2 tsp Salt
- 2 tsp Spicy Brown Mustard
- 1 Tbsp + 1 tsp Erythritol
- 1 Tbsp Red Wine Vinegar

---

[17] Eat This Much, I. (2019). *Eat This Much, your personal diet assistant.* [online] Eat This Much. Available at: https://www.eatthismuch.com/recipe/nutrition/keto-szechuan-chicken,955690/ [Accessed 25 Feb. 2019].

Direction

1. Mix tomato paste, soy sauce, chili garlic paste, brown mustard, and ginger together inside a ramekin.

2. Bring 3 Tbsp of coconut oil to medium-high temperature on the stove.

3. Cook the ground chicken using pepper and salt in the oil until it is thoroughly cooked. Break all of it up into small pieces.

4. Pour 2/3 of your sauce inside the mixture and mix it thoroughly.

5. Include the spinach with your chicken and allow it to wilt. Pour salt, pepper, Mrs. Dash seasoning, and also red pepper flakes.

6. Add the remaining 1/3 of your sauce, chicken stock, red wine vinegar, and also erythritol. Mix up the spinach and spices in thoroughly.

7. Turn the heat to low and then cover the pan. Allow this to cook for about 10- 15 minutes.

Not Your Caveman's Chili

Yields 4 Total Servings, per serving, this is 5.3g Net Carbs, 17.8g Fats, 51.8g Protein and 398 Calories. (Freeze Leftovers)[18]

Ingredients

1 tsp Worcestershire

1 tsp Cayenne Pepper

1 tsp Oregano

2 tsp Paprika

2 tsp Minced Garlic

2 tsp Red Boat Fish Sauce

1 Medium Green Pepper

2 lbs. Stew Meat

1/3 Cup Tomato Paste

1 Medium Onion

1 Cup Beef Broth

2 Tbsp + 1 tsp Chili Powder

2 Tbsp Olive Oil

2 Tbsp Soy Sauce

1 1/2 tsp Cumin

---

[18] KD Recipes. (2019). *Modified Not Your Caveman's Chili*. [online] Available at: https://kdrecipesblog.wordpress.com/2017/09/08/modified-not-your-Caveman's-chili/ [Accessed 25 Feb. 2019].

Direction

1. Cube half of the stew meat into small cubes, then process the remaining portion inside a food processor into ground beef.

2. Chop up the pepper and onion into small pieces.

3. Combine all of the spices together to prepare the sauce.

4. Sauté beef that is cubed in a pan until browned, then transfer it to a slow cooker. Do likewise with the ground beef.

5. Sauté the vegetables in the fat that is left in the pan until onions turn lucid.

6. Add all of it to the slow cooker and mix it all up.

7. On high, simmer for 2 1/2 hours, then simmer for about 20-30 minutes in the absence of the top.

Omnivore Burger with Roasted Almonds & Creamed Spinach

Yields 2 total Servings, each coming out to 4.8g Net Carbs, 38.5g Fats, 45.3g Protein and 562 Calories.[19]

Ingredients

- 100g (~1 Cup) Sliced Mushrooms
- 1/4 Bell Pepper
- Pound Ground Beef
- 1/4 Onion 1
- 2 1/2 Tbsp Roasted Almonds
- 2 1/2 Cups Raw Spinach
- 1 tsp Red Pepper Flakes
- 1 Tbsp Cream Cheese
- 1/2 Tbsp Tone's Southwest Chipotle Seasoning 1 tsp Cumin
- 1/2 Tbsp Butter
- 1/2 Tbsp Heavy Cream

---

[19] OneEarthHealth. (2019). *Omnivore Burger with Creamed Spinach and Roasted Almonds*. [online] Available at: https://oneearthhealth.com/blogs/keto-recipes/omnivore-burger-with-creamed-spinach-and-roasted-almonds [Accessed 25 Feb. 2019].

Direction

1. Preheat your oven until it reaches 450 convection or 475 normal. (Convection is preferable)

2. Measure out a 100g portion of mushrooms, 1/4 onion, and 1/4 bell pepper. Put them inside the food processor and continue to pulse until you get diced vegetables.

3. Pour your meat, diced vegetables, and seasonings inside a bowl used for mixing and mix thoroughly.

4. From the meat, make a portion of 3 burger patties.

5. On a cooling rack that is sitting over a baking sheet, rest the 3 patties. The sheet for baking ought to be covered in foil and salt added to it (to catch the drippings).

6. Put little measure of what is left of the meat into a pan and allow to sizzle.

7. Add spinach to it and allow it to wilt with some salt, pepper, and red pepper flakes as well.

8. Pour in almonds, cream cheese, butter, heavy cream and mix it up thoroughly. Allow it to continue to cook down and remain warm.

9. After 19-24 minutes, take the burgers away from the oven. Ensure that you keep your eye on these because once they begin to get past the temperature for being rare, they begin to cook rapidly.

10.

Bacon Wrapped Pork Tenderloin

This makes 1 total serving with leftovers. This comes out to 0.3g Net Carbs, 20g Fats, 54g Protein and 418 Calories.[20]

Ingredients

- Pinch Dried Sage
- Pinch Black Pepper
- Pinch Cayenne
- 3/4 tsp Soy Sauce
- 1/4 tsp Dried Rosemary
- 1/4 tsp Liquid Smoke
- 1/4 tsp Minced Garlic
- 2 1/2 Slices Bacon
- 1/2 lb. Pork Tenderloin
- 1 1/2 tsp Sugar-Free Maple Syrup
- 1 1/2 tsp Dijon Mustard

Direction

1. Mix all of the wet and dry ingredients together to prepare the marinated mixture.

2. Dry pat the pork tenderloins then add them into a

---

[20] Tenderloin, B. (2019). *Bacon Wrapped Pork Tenderloin | Ruled Me*. [online] Ruled Me. Available at: https://www.ruled.me/bacon-wrapped-pork-tenderloin/ [Accessed 25 Feb. 2019].

Ziploc bag.

3. Pour the marinade into a bag and rub it onto the tenderloins. Place this inside the fridge for a period of 3-5 hours.

4. Preheat your oven to a temperature of 350F.

5. Place the pork tenderloins on a foiled sheet for baking, then wrap it up in bacon. It should be about 5 slices per tenderloin.

6. Bake for 60 minutes, after this broil, the bacon for about 5-10 minutes.

7. Cover the tenderloins up with foil for about 10-15 minutes to rest. After this cut it up and serve.

Red Pepper Spinach Salad

This makes 1 total serving. This comes out to 3.5g Net Carbs, 18g Fats, 8g Protein and 208 Calories.[21]

Ingredients

- 1/2 tsp Red Pepper Flakes
- 1 1/2 Tbsp Parmesan Cheese
- 2 Tbsp Ranch Dressing
- 3 Cups Spinach

Direction

1. Add spinach into a bowl used for mixing, after this drench in ranch.
2. Mix everything up together and then add your parmesan and red pepper flakes.
3. Mix everything once again and then serve.

---

[21] Salad, R. (2019). *Red Pepper Spinach Salad | Ruled Me*. [online] Ruled Me. Available at: https://www.ruled.me/red-pepper-spinach-salad/ [Accessed 25 Feb. 2019].

Roasted Pecan Green Beans

This makes 3 total servings. Per serving this is 3.3g Net Carbs, 16.8g Fats, 3.7g Protein and 182 Calories. (Freeze Leftovers)[22]

Ingredients

- 2 Tbsp Olive Oil
- 1/2 Pound Green Beans
- 2 Tbsp Parmesan Cheese
- 1/4 Cup Chopped Pecans
- 1/2 tsp Red Pepper Flakes
- 1 tsp Minced Garlic
- 1/2 Lemon Zest

Direction

1. Preheat oven to a temperature of 450F, after this add pecans to your food processor.
2. Continue to grind the pecans inside the food processor until everything is nicely chopped. A few pieces should be large, some should be small.
3. Make a mixture of green beans, pecans, olive oil, parmesan cheese, 1/2 lemon zest, garlic that has been minced, and red pepper flakes inside a large bowl used for mixing.

---

[22] Keto Carlo. (2019). *ROASTED PECAN GREEN BEANS*. [online] Available at: https://www.ketocarlo.com/roasted-pecan-green-beans.html [Accessed 25 Feb. 2019].

4. Spread the green beans out on the foiled sheet used for baking.

5. Roast the green beans inside your oven for a period of 20-25 minutes.

6. Allow it to cool for a period of 4-5 minutes, then serve after this!

Shrimp & Cauliflower Curry

This gives 6 total servings. Each serving comes out to 5.6g Net Carbs, 19.5g Fats, 27.4g Protein and 331 Calories. (Freeze Leftovers)[23]

Double the serving size If you're on week 2.

Ingredients

- 1/4 tsp Xanthan Gum
- 1/4 tsp Cinnamon
- 1/4 tsp Cardamom
- 1/2 tsp Coriander
- 1/2 tsp Ground Ginger
- 1/2 tsp Turmeric
- 1 tsp Paprika
- 1 tsp Chili Powder
- 1 tsp Cayenne
- 1 tsp Onion powder
- 24 Oz. Shrimp
- 5 Cups Raw Spinach
- 3 Tbsp Olive Oil

---

[23] Keto Carlo. (2019). *SHRIMP & CAULIFLOWER CURRY*. [online] Available at: https://www.ketocarlo.com/shrimp--cauliflower-curry.html [Accessed 25 Feb. 2019].

- 2 tsp Garlic Powder
- 2 Tbsp Curry Powder
- 1 Tbsp Cumin
- 1 Tbsp Coconut Flour
- 1/4 Cup Butter
- 1/2 Head Medium Cauliflower
- 4 Cups Chicken Stock
- 1 Cup Coconut Milk
- 1 Medium Onion
- 1/4 Cup Heavy Cream

Direction

1. Mix up all spices (with the exception of xanthan and coconut flour), and put it aside.
2. Cut up a medium sized onion into slices.
3. Inside a pan, bring 3 Tbsp of olive oil to hot heat. Add the onion and cook till its soft.
4. Add butter, heavy cream, 1/8 tsp of spices and xanthan, stir it in so it's all thoroughly mixed.
5. Add 4 cups of chicken broth, and a cup of coconut milk after about 1-2 minutes of the spices sweating. Stir thoroughly and cover.
6. Cook for about 30 minutes, with the lid on the pot. Chop up cauliflower into small florets then add it to curry. While it is still covered, cook for an additional

15 minutes.

7. Detail and devein the shrimp, then add the shrimp to the curry. With the lid off, cook for an extra 20 minutes.

8. Measure out coconut flour and 1/8 tsp of xanthan gum and stir it thoroughly into the curry. Allow it to cook for 5 minutes.

9. After 5 minutes have passed, add spinach and mix it in thoroughly. With the lid off, cook for an extra 5-10 minutes.

Simple Lunch Salad

This makes 1 total serving. Macros are dependent on the type of meat you eat.

Ingredients

- Meat Specified in Day-by-Day
- Zest 1/4 Lemon
- 1 1/2 tsp Dijon Mustard
- 1 Tbsp - 2 Tbsp Parmesan Cheese
- 3/4 tsp Curry Powder (optional)
- 2 Cups Spinach
- 2 Tbsp - 4 Tbsp Olive Oil

Direction

1. Make a combination of all wet ingredients inside a small bowl.
2. Make a combination of meat and spinach in a bowl.
3. When you are ready to eat, pour wet ingredients over the meat and spinach.

Keto Snickerdoodle Cookies

Yields 14 total cookies. One cookie is 2g Net Carbs, 12.4g Fats, 3.4g Protein and 132 Calories.[24]

Ingredients

- 2 Tbsp Cinnamon
- 2 Cups Almond Flour
- 1/4 Cup Maple Syrup
- 1/4 Cup Coconut Oil
- 1/4 tsp Baking Soda
- 1 Tbsp Vanilla

Direction

1. Preheat oven to a temperature of 350F.
2. Mix your almond flour, baking soda, and salt together.
3. Make a mixture of coconut oil, homemade maple syrup, vanilla, and stevia in a separate bowl.
4. Continue to mix dry ingredients into wet ingredients until a dough is formed.
5. Continue to mix cinnamon and erythritol together until a powder is formed.

---

[24] Keto Carlo. (2019). *KETO SNICKERDOODLE COOKIES*. [online] Available at: https://www.ketocarlo.com/keto-snickerdoodle-cookies.html [Accessed 25 Feb. 2019].

6. Roll the dough into balls, roll them into cinnamon mixture. After this, set them on a silpat.

7. To flatten out the balls, utilize a mason jar underside greasing the base as required.

8. Bake for a period of 9-10 minutes, take it off and allow it to cool.

Low Carb Spice Cakes

This makes 12 total frosted cakes. For each frosted cake, they are: 3.3g Carbs, 27g Fats, 7.3g Protein and 283 Calories.[25]

Ingredients

- 1/2 tsp Nutmeg
- 1/2 tsp Cinnamon
- 1/2 tsp Ginger
- 2 Cups Honeyville Almond Flour
- Spice Cakes
- 1/4 tsp Ground Clove
- 1/2 tsp Allspice
- 1/2 Cup Salted Butter
- 1 tsp Vanilla Extract
- 2 tsp Baking Powder
- 5 Tbsp Water
- 4 Large Eggs
- 3/4 Cup Erythritol

Cream Cheese Frosting

- 1/2 of Lemon Zest

---

[25] Keto Carlo. (2019). *LOW CARB SPICE CAKES*. [online] Available at: https://www.ketocarlo.com/low-carb-spice-cakes.html [Accessed 25 Feb. 2019].

- 2 Tbsp Butter

- 8 Oz. Cream Cheese

- 3 Tbsp Erythritol

- 1 tsp Vanilla Extract

Direction

1. Preheat your oven to a temperature of 350F.

2. Add your butter and sweetener inside a bowl used for mixing. Continue to cream it together until smooth.

3. Add 2 of your eggs and keep on mixing it until combined, add and mix in your last 2 eggs after this.

4. Grind your spices, after this add all the dry ingredients to the batter. Mix until it is smooth.

5. Continue to add your water to the batter and mix thoroughly until it becomes creamy.

6. Spray your cupcake tray and fill it up to about 3/4, then place them inside the oven for about 15 minutes.

7. While they are still cooking, cream your cream cheese, butter, sweetener, vanilla, and lemon zest together for the icing.

8. Take your cupcakes away from the oven, allow them to cool for 15 minutes, then ice them.

Chicken and Bacon Sausage Stir Fry

This makes 3 total servings. For each serving, it is: 7.3g Net Carbs, 28.3g Fats, 35.7g Protein and 451 Calories. (Freeze Leftovers)[26]

Ingredients

- 3 Cups Spinach
- 1/2 Cup Rao's Tomato Sauce
- 1/2 Cup Parmesan Cheese
- 1/2 tsp Red Pepper Flakes
- 4 Chicken Sausages
- 3 Cups Broccoli Florets
- 1/4 Cup Red Wine
- 2 tsp Minced Garlic
- 2 Tbsp Salted Butter

Direction

1. Slice up the 4 pieces of bacon & cheddar chicken sausages.
2. Begin to boil water on the stove. Add your sausage to

---

[26] Fry, C. (2019). *Chicken and Bacon Sausage Stir Fry | Ruled Me*. [online] Ruled Me. Available at: https://www.ruled.me/chicken-bacon-sausage-stir-fry/ [Accessed 25 Feb. 2019].

a pan that is on high heat while this is going on.

3. Add your broccoli to the water that is being boiled and cook for about 3-5 minutes dependent on how you like it done.

4. Continue to stir your sausages until they become brown on the two sides.

5. Move the sausages to a side of the pan, and add the butter to it. Put your garlic in the butter and allow it to sauté for 60 seconds.

6. Mix everything together thoroughly and then add your broccoli to it.

7. Pour in the tomato sauce, red wine, then pour the red pepper flakes.

8. Make a mixture of these, pour in your spinach with salt and pepper, then allow it to cool down. Let this simmer for about 5-10 minutes.

Taco Tartlets

This makes 11 total tartlets. Each tartlet have: 1.7g Net Carbs, 19.4g Fats, 13.1g Protein and 241 Calories. (Freeze All Leftovers, Use as Snacks- We Do Not Use Them Anymore)[27]

Ingredients

The Pastry

- 1/4 tsp Salt
- 1 tsp Oregano
- 1 tsp Xanthan Gum
- 1/4 tsp Cayenne
- 1/4 tsp Paprika
- 1 Cup Blanched Almond Flour
- 5 Tbsp Butter
- 3 Tbsp Coconut Flour
- 2 Tbsp Ice Water

The Filling

- 1/4 tsp Cinnamon
- 1 tsp Worcestershire
- 400g Ground Beef

---

[27] Tartlets, L. (2019). *Low Carb Taco Tartlets | Ruled Me*. [online] Ruled Me. Available at: https://www.ruled.me/low-carb-taco-tartlets/ [Accessed 25 Feb. 2019].

- 1 tsp Salt
- 1/2 tsp Pepper
- 1/3 Cup Cheese
- 3 Stalks Spring Onion
- 2 tsp Yellow Mustard
- 1 tsp Cumin
- 80g Mushroom
- 1 Tbsp Olive Oil
- 2 Tbsp Tomato Paste
- 2 tsp Garlic

Direction

1. Combine each of the pastry's dry ingredients and place them inside a food processor.

2. Chop up cold butter into little square shapes then add it to the food processor as well. Pulse the dough together until it is crumbly, keep adding 1 Tbsp of ice water until pliable.

3. Chill your dough inside the freezer for about 10 minutes.

4. Using a rolling pin, roll out the dough between 2 silpats. With a cookie cutter or a glass, cut out circles.

5. Place the dough inside your whoopie pan and preheat your oven to a temperature of 325F.

6. Prepare all the ingredients for filling – chop the spring onions, mince the garlic, and slice the mushrooms.

7. Sauté the onions and garlic inside olive oil. Add your ground beef into this mixture and then sear it well – adding the dry spices and Worcestershire as well.

8. pour the mushrooms and mix them together thoroughly. Then right before finishing, add tomato paste and mustard.

9. Add ground beef mixture in an even manner into the pastry tartlets. Cover it with cheese and proceed to bake for about 20-25 minutes.

10. This is Optional: Before you take out the oven, broil for about 3-5 minutes.

11. Let it cool completely and take the pastries away.

Thai Peanut Chicken

This makes 2 total servings. For each serving, it is: 8.8g Net Carbs, 53.5g Fats, 70.5g Protein and 743 Calories. (Freeze Leftovers[28]

Ingredients

- 2 tsp Chili Garlic Paste
- 1/4 tsp Cayenne Pepper
- 1/4 tsp Coriander
- Salt + Pepper to taste
- 1 Tbsp Rice Vinegar
- 1 Tbsp Orange Juice
- 1/2 tsp Sesame Oil
- 1/2 Tbsp Coconut Oil
- 6 Boneless, Skinless Chicken Thighs
- 1 Tbsp Lemon Juice
- 1 Cup Peanuts (1/2 Cup Peanut Butter if you aren't making your own)
- 1/2 Tbsp Erythritol
- 2 Tbsp Soy Sauce
- 1/4 Cup Chicken Stock

---

[28] Allrecipes. (2019). *Thai Peanut Chicken Recipe*. [online] Available at: https://www.allrecipes.com/recipe/50658/thai-peanut-chicken/ [Accessed 25 Feb. 2019].

Direction

1. To dispose extra moisture, rinse peanuts off and spin them inside a salad spinner. Pat it dry using paper towels.

2. Put the nuts inside your food processor and blend them until they become creamy. Add coconut oil and erythritol then blend further.

3. Mix all of the ingredients together with the exception of salt and pepper to prepare your sauce.

4. Cube the thighs of your chicken and season them using salt and pepper.

5. In a pan, heat a Tbsp of olive oil to high heat. Once it is hot, add your chicken.

6. With a paper towel, pat the extra moisture out of the pan. Until the chicken is browned on two sides, continue to cook.

7. Pour in your peanut butter sauce, then add 1/4 tsp of cayenne pepper. add extra pepper and salt if you so desire.

8. Turn to low and allow it to simmer for about 10 minutes.

Vanilla Latte Cookies

Makes 10 total cookies. For each cookie, they are: 1.4g Net Carbs, 17.1g Fats, 3.9g Protein and 167 Calories.[29]

Ingredients

- 17 Drops Liquid Stevia
- 2 Large Eggs
- 1 Tbsp + 1 tsp Instant Coffee Grounds
- 1 1/2 Cups Honeyville Blanched Almond Flour 1/2 Cup Unsalted Butter 1/3 Cup NOW Erythritol
- 1 1/2 tsp Vanilla Extract
- 1/2 tsp Kosher Salt
- 1/2 tsp Baking Soda
- 1/4 tsp Cinnamon
- 17 Drops Liquid Stevia

Direction

1. Preheat your oven to a temperature of 350F.
2. Make a combination of your almond flour, coffee grounds, baking soda, salt, and cinnamon inside a mixing bowl

---

[29] Anon, (2019). [online] Available at: http://sugarcrafter.net/2011/11/03/vanilla-latte-cookies/ [Accessed 25 Feb. 2019].

3. Separate your egg whites and egg yolks in different containers or bowls

4. Add your butter and beat it thoroughly inside a separate mixing bowl. Add your erythritol to the butter and keep on beating it until it is almost white.

5. Add the yolk of your eggs to the butter and continue to mix until it is smooth.

6. Add one half of your mixed almond flour to the butter and mix it well. Pour your vanilla extract and liquid stevia too, after this add what is left of your almond flour and mix thoroughly.

7. Continue to beat your egg whites until stiff peaks are formed. Fold up the egg whites into the cookie dough.

8. On a cookie sheet, divide your cookies, I prepared 10 big cookies. Bake them for about 12-15 minutes.

9. Remove the cookies to a cooling rack for 10-15 minutes once it is done.

Vegetable Medley

This makes 3 servings. For each serving, it is: 7.7g Net Carbs, 30.7g Fats, 6.7g Protein and 330 Calories.

Ingredients

- 90g Spinach
- 90g Bell Pepper
- 1 tsp Salt
- 1/2 tsp Red Pepper Flakes
- 240g Baby Bella Mushrooms
- 2 tsp Minced Garlic
- 2 Tbsp Pumpkin Seeds
- 6 Tbsp Olive Oil
- 100g Sugar Snap Peas
- 115g Broccoli
- 1 tsp Pepper

Direction

1. Prepare all the vegetables by chopping them into small, bite-size pieces.
2. In a pan, heat oil to high heat. Add garlic and let it sauté for 60 seconds once it is hot.

3. Add mushrooms and allow them to soak up part of the oil. Add broccoli and mix together once this happens.

4. Allow broccoli to cook for some minutes, after this pour in your sugar snap peas. Mix everything together thoroughly.

5. Add the spices, bell pepper, and pumpkin seeds. After this mix together thoroughly.

6. Lay the spinach over the vegetables and allow them to steam wilt it once everything is cooked.

7. Once the spinach has wilted, mix everything together and serve.

Chapter 8. Ketogenic Smoothie Recipes

Shopping List

The ingredients from every smoothie recipe in this section makes up the below shopping list. You may decide to get every item on the list to save them on hand so when you desire to have something different, you can also vary your smoothies daily. This gives you a high daily smoothie motivation and your desired result!

Fruit

- Raspberries (fresh or frozen)
- Wild Blueberries (frozen)
- Banana (may freeze when browning)
- Pineapple (frozen)
- Mangos (frozen)

Dairy-Free Nut Milk

- Unsweetened Vanilla Coconut Milk
- Unsweetened Vanilla Almond Milk

Vegetables

- Spinach (fresh or frozen)
- Kale (fresh or frozen)
- Ginger
- Chard (fresh or frozen)

Miscellaneous

- Flax or chia seeds
- 1 Tbsp Coconut Oil/Cream

Chocolate Almond Smoothie[30]

instead of using almond butter and almond milk, use coconut butter and coconut milk to turn this into a chocolate coconut smoothie.

Ingredients

Serves two

- ¼ cup sugar-free almond butter
- 1 cup unsweetened almond milk
- ¼ cup heavy cream
- 2 Tbsp s unsweetened cocoa powder
- 5 drops liquid stevia (optional)
- 1½ cups ice

Directions

1. Place all the ingredients to be used in a blender and blend until it's smooth.
2. Serve chilled.

---

[30] Primaltoad.com. (2019). *Low Carb Chocolate Almond Smoothie – Primal Toad*. [online] Available at: https://primaltoad.com/low-carb-chocolate-almond-smoothie/ [Accessed 5 Mar. 2019].

Pumpkin Pie Smoothie

Don't get confused, canned pumpkin pie filling is different from pumpkin purée, people confuse these two. pumpkin pie filling is made up of sweeteners that increase carbohydrate and sugar content, while Pure pumpkin purée is made up of only the flesh of a pumpkin.

Ingredients[31]

Serves two

- 1 cup full-fat canned coconut milk
- 1/2 cup pumpkin purée
- 1/4 large avocado
- 1/2 tsp pumpkin pie spice
- 1/4 tsp maple extract
- 2 Tbsp s coconut oil, melted
- 1/4 cup unsweetened whey protein powder

Directions

1. Put all the ingredients to be used in a blender and blend until it's smooth.
2. Serve chilled.

---

[31] Liv Breathe Keto. (2019). *Pumpkin Pie Protein Shake – Liv Breathe Keto*. [online] Available at: https://livbreatheketo.com/pumpkin-pie-protein-shake/ [Accessed 5 Mar. 2019].

Green Smoothie

For this recipe, the chosen whey protein powder type will bring about a big difference in the taste. To switch it up, alternate between vanilla and chocolate.

Ingredients[32][33]

Serves two

- ½ tsp vanilla extract
- 2 drops liquid stevia
- ½ cup baby spinach
- ½ avocado
- 1 cup full-fat canned coconut milk
- ¼ cup whey protein powder

Directions

1. Put all the ingredients to be used in a blender and blend until it's smooth.
2. Serve immediately.

---

[32] Simple Green Smoothies. (2019). *The BEST Green Smoothie Recipe Ever | Simple Green Smoothies.* [online] Available at: https://simplegreensmoothies.com/recipes/beginners-luck-green-smoothie [Accessed 5 Mar. 2019].

[33] *Keto Green Smoothie - 4g net carbs - Ditch The Carbs.* (2019). [online] Ditch The Carbs. Available at: https://www.ditchthecarbs.com/keto-green-smoothie/ [Accessed 5 Mar. 2019].

Honeydew and Avocado Smoothie

This sweet and creamy smoothie combines plenty of healthy fats and protein to keep you full and strong the whole day. Try using a slightly different flavor instead of cantaloupe or your favorite melon.

Ingredients[34][35]

Serves one

- 2 Tbsp s unsweetened whey protein powder
- 1/4 medium avocado, peeled and pit removed
- 1/2 cup full-fat canned coconut milk
- 1/4 cup chunks honeydew melon
- 1 Tbsp chia seeds
- 1/4 cup water
- Ice, to thicken, if desired

---

[34] *Hass Avocado Honeydew Smoothie Recipe* .(2019) [online] Hispanic Kitchen. Available at: https://hispanickitchen.com/recipes/hass-avocado-honeydew-smoothie-recipe/ [Accessed 5 Mar. 2019].
[35] Lindsey Janeiro, C. (2019). *Honeydew Avocado Kale Smoothie | Nutrition to Fit*. [online] Nutrition to Fit. Available at: https://nutritiontofit.com/honeydew-avocado-kale-smoothie/ [Accessed 5 Mar. 2019].

Directions

1. Put coconut milk, melon, avocado, protein powder, chia seeds, and water in a blender and blend until it's smooth.
2. to thicken, Add ice. (if desired)
3. Serve chilled.

Carrot Asparagus Green Smoothie

flaxseed, when added to this smoothie, boosts the mineral and vitamin content, also gives a delicious hint of nutty flavor.

Ingredients[36]

Serves four

- 1 cup water
- 2 cups full-fat canned coconut milk
- 1 cup chopped asparagus
- 1 cup watercress
- 2 Tbsp s flaxseed
- 2 small carrots, peeled and chopped

Directions

1. Combine flaxseed, coconut milk, carrots, asparagus, and watercress in a blender, blend until it's well combined.
2. While blending, Add water until a desired texture is achieved.

---

[36] Magary, V. (2019). *How To Make A Green Smoothie / Ultimate Paleo Guide*. [online] Ultimate Paleo Guide. Available at: https://ultimatepaleoguide.com/make-green-smoothie/ [Accessed 5 Mar. 2019].

Avocado Raspberry Smoothie

This smoothie is sweet and satisfying, makes a good breakfast. For a more exotic touch, Try substituting the raspberries with blackberries, blueberries, or even cloudberries.

Ingredients[37][38]

Serves 1

- ½ cup water
- 2 Tbsp s coconut oil, melted
- ¼ cup raspberries
- ¼ medium avocado, peeled and pit removed
- 1 cup heavy cream
- ½ cup chopped fresh mint

Directions

1. Put mint, coconut oil, cream, raspberries, and avocado in a blender and blend until smooth.
2. While blending, Add water until you get a desired consistency.

---

[37] *Raspberry Avocado Smoothie - Dairy Free.* (2019). [online] Low Carb Yum. Available at: https://lowcarbyum.com/raspberry-avocado-smoothie-low-carb/ [Accessed 5 Mar. 2019].

[38] *Raspberry and Avocado Smoothie | Nadia Lim.*(2019). [online] Nadia Lim. Available at: https://nadialim.com/recipe/raspberry-avocado-smoothie/ [Accessed 5 Mar. 2019].

Triple Green Smoothie

This smoothie features avocado, lime, and spinach for a balance of flavors, and a boost of vitamins and whole nutrition. try swapping away spinach for watercress or romaine lettuce If the taste is too strong for your palate.

Ingredients[39]

Serves four

- 1 cup full-fat coconut milk
- 1 cup fresh spinach
- 1 large lime, peeled and seeded
- 2 medium avocados, peeled and pits removed
- 3⁄4 cup full-fat plain Greek yogurt

Directions

1. Combine 1⁄2 cup coconut milk, spinach, lime, 1⁄2 cup yogurt, and avocados in a blender and blend until it is well combined.

2. While blending, Add remaining 1⁄2 cup yogurt and 1⁄2 cup coconut milk until a desired texture is achieved.

---

[39] IdealFit. (2019). *Triple Green Smoothie | IdealFit*. [online] Available at: https://www.idealfit.com/blog/triple-green-smoothie/ [Accessed 5 Mar. 2019].

Almond Berry Smoothie

This flavorful smoothie is graced by Almonds—whole almonds and almond butter combine for a mix of smooth and crunchy textures. The addition of flaxseed (which even adds nuttier flavor) boosts the omega-3 content of this smoothie.

Ingredients[40]

Serves four

- 1/2 cup heavy cream
- 1 cup strawberries
- 2 cups unsweetened homemade almond milk, divided (see sidebar in Banana Nut Smoothie recipe)
- 1/4 cup raw almonds
- 2 Tbsp s unsweetened almond butter
- 1 cup fresh spinach
- 1 Tbsp flaxseed

Directions

1. Combine 1 cup almond milk with the almonds, flaxseed, and almond butter in a blender and emulsify. Emulsify completely until no nut pieces is remaining For a smoother texture, For a chunky texture, leave some pieces of almond intact.

---

[40] Foodnetwork.com. (2019). *Best Almond Milk And Berry Smoothie recipes.* [online] Available at: https://www.foodnetwork.com/recipes/melissa-darabian/almond-milk-and-berry-smoothie-recipe-1960870 [Accessed 5 Mar. 2019].

2. Add heavy cream, spinach, and strawberries, blend until it is well combined.

3. While blending, Add the remaining 1 cup of almond milk as required until your desired consistency is reached.

Kale and Brazil Nut Smoothie

This is an unusual blend of ingredients which gives a unique flavor and sound nutrition . Kale is known as a nutritional powerhouse which provides vitamins A and K in abundance.

About 91% of Brazil nuts' calories is from fat, this makes them a perfect to add to the ketogenic diet.

Ingredients[41]

Serves 2

- 1/2–1 cup ice, as needed
- 1/2 tsp ground allspice
- 1/4 cup Brazil nuts, frozen
- 2 cups chopped kale
- 2 cups full-fat canned coconut milk
- 2 Tbsp s coconut oil, melted
- 1/2 tsp ground cinnamon

Directions

1. Place cinnamon, coconut oil, kale, coconut milk, nuts, and allspice in a blender, blend until it is well combined.
2. With the blender running, add ice bits by bits until you reach a desired consistency. Add splashes of water If the smoothie is too thick to thin out the consistency.

---

[41] Kale and Brazil Nut Smoothie, (2019). [online] Available at: https://www.kroger.com/r/kale-brazil-nut-smoothie-recipe/175389 [Accessed 5 Mar. 2019].

Calming Cucumber Smoothie

The refreshing fragrance of mint and the light taste of cucumber in combination with romaine lettuce makes this smoothie delightful. A great addition to this smoothie is toasted almonds; in addition to the coconut flakes, try adding a tablespoon of sliced toasted almonds.

Ingredients

[42]Serves four

- ¼ cup chopped mint
- ¼ cup unsweetened coconut flakes
- 2 medium cucumbers, peeled
- 1 cup chopped romaine lettuce
- 1 cup full-fat canned coconut milk, divided

Directions

1. Combine ½ cup coconut milk, cucumbers, romaine, and mint thoroughly in a blender.
2. While blending, add the remaining coconut milk.
3. The smoothie mixture should be divided into 4 glasses, with each glass Topped with 1 tablespoon coconut flakes to garnish.

---

[42] *Cucumber Spinach Smoothie | Ruled Me.*(2019) [online] Ruled Me. Available at: https://www.ruled.me/cucumber-spinach-smoothie/ [Accessed 5 Mar. 2019].

Spiced Cashew Butter Smoothie

Substitute the usual almond butter– and peanut butter–filled smoothies with cashew butter instead! Cashew butter is very creamy and slightly sweet. The best is raw cashew butter, it has higher levels of nutrients than the roasted one.

Ingredients[43][44]

Serves one

- 1 tsp crushed cashews (optional)
- ½ cup ice
- ½ tsp ground cinnamon
- ½ cup heavy cream
- 1 Tbsp unsweetened cashew butter
- ½ avocado, peeled and pit removed
- ½ cup full-fat canned coconut milk
- ½ tsp sugar-free vanilla extract
- ½ tsp ground allspice

Directions

---

[43] *Banana Cashew Butter Chia Seed Smoothie - Jar Of Lemons.*(2019) [online] Jar Of Lemons. Available at: https://www.jaroflemons.com/banana-cashew-butter-chia-seed-smoothie/ [Accessed 5 Mar. 2019].

[44] *Chai Spiced Cashew Butter & Froothie Optimum 9400 Review - Domestic Gothess.*(2019) [online] Available at: https://domesticgothess.com/blog/2018/01/24/chai-spiced-cashew-butter/ [Accessed 5 Mar. 2019].

1. Combine cashew heavy cream, vanilla extract, coconut milk, cinnamon, butter, avocado, and allspice in a blender and thoroughly combine.

2. While blending, add ice slowly until you reach the desired texture.

3. Pour the mixture into a glass and top with 1 teaspoon of crushed cashews, if desired.

Spiced Chocolate Smoothie

Without all the added carbohydrates and sugar the traditional version of Mexican hot chocolate contains; this smoothie contains flavors that are reminiscent to it—. Skip cayenne powder from this smoothie if it's too spicy for your taste buds. Instead, Try putting a pinch of nutmeg.

Ingredients[45]

Serves one

- 1 cinnamon stick, to garnish
- 1/2 cup ice, if desired
- 1 Tbsp coconut oil, melted
- 1/2 cup full-fat canned coconut milk
- 1/4 tsp cayenne powder
- 1 Tbsp ground flaxseed or chia seeds
- 2 1/2 Tbsp s unsweetened cocoa powder
- 1/2 tsp ground cinnamon
- 1/2 cup water
- 1/4 tsp unsweetened vanilla extract

---

[45] *Oaxaca Chocolate Banana Smoothie Recipe - Cookie and Kate* .(2019) [online] Cookie and Kate. Available at: https://cookieandkate.com/2013/oaxaca-chocolate-banana-smoothie/ [Accessed 5 Mar. 2019].

Directions

1. Combine cinnamon, vanilla extract, coconut milk, ground seeds, coconut oil, water, cocoa powder, and cayenne in a blender and thoroughly combine.

2. While blending, add ice slowly until desired texture is gotten.

3. Pour the smoothie mixture into a glass and garnish with cinnamon stick, if desired.

Orange Coconut Smoothie

This smoothie is packed with immune-system-boosting and brain-stimulating vitamin C, it is a great option when it seems everyone around you is sick. The antioxidant-rich coconut milk intensifies Its power.

Ingredients[46] [47]

Serves 4

- 2 tablespoons coconut oil, melted
- 2 cups full-fat canned coconut milk
- 2 medium oranges, peeled
- 1 cup chopped iceberg lettuce

Directions

1. Blend oranges and lettuce until well combined.
2. While blending, slowly Add coconut oil and coconut milk until a desired consistency is achieved.

---

[46] Day, R. (2019). *Coconut-Orange Smoothie*. [online] Rachael Ray Every Day. Available at: https://www.rachaelraymag.com/recipe/coconut-orange-smoothie [Accessed 5 Mar. 2019].

[47] *Creamy Orange Coconut Smoothie | Occasionally Eggs* .(2019) [online] Occasionally Eggs. Available at: https://www.occasionallyeggs.com/creamy-orange-coconut-smoothie/ [Accessed 5 Mar. 2019].

Banana-Lettuce Smoothie

In this smoothie, there is a combination of the healthy fats and ample protein that you need. In addition to the minerals, vitamins, and nutrients from the banana and lettuce, the coconut milk has some healthy fats which makes this smoothie a strong start to any day.

Ingredients[48] [49] [50]

Serves 4

- 1 medium banana, sliced
- 1 cup homemade unsweetened vanilla almond milk
- 1 cup chopped iceberg lettuce
- 1 cup full-fat canned coconut milk
- ½ tsp vanilla extract
- 1 cup heavy cream

---

[48] Tri-Wellness. (2019). *Banana Berry Lettuce Smoothie - Tri-Wellness*. [online] Available at: https://lisashanken.com/recipe/banana-berry-lettuce-smoothie/ [Accessed 5 Mar. 2019].
[49] Banana, G. (2019). *Green Smoothie: Romaine Lettuce & Banana Recipe*. [online] SparkRecipes. Available at: https://recipes.sparkpeople.com/recipe-detail.asp?recipe=1581664 [Accessed 5 Mar. 2019].
[50] Creme De La Crumb. (2019). *Banana Nut Smoothie Bowl | Creme De La Crumb*. [online] Available at: https://www.lecremedelacrumb.com/banana-nut-smoothie-bowl/ [Accessed 5 Mar. 2019].

Directions

1. Combine lettuce, vanilla extract, heavy cream, and coconut milk in a blender with half cup of almond milk and thoroughly blend.

2. While blending, keep adding remaining almond milk until you reach a desired consistency.

3. Divide smoothie into 4 glasses. each glass should be topped with an equal amount of sliced banana.

Keto-Friendly Snacks

If during the day, you begin to feel hungry at any point, always keep some keto friendly snacks handy. You are not supposed to get hungry between meals, but you sometimes do in the initial stages of your ketogenic diet, you need a little time to adjust. Here are some keto-friendly snacks that can be of help!

- Sugar-free Jello
- Pickles
- Nuts (pecans, walnuts, macadamias, brazil nuts)
- Pork rinds – perfect with about just anything
- Nut butters –almond, peanut, coconut, cashew, etc. Be sure no sugar is added.
- Sardines –add some Old Bay seasoning!
- Laughing Cow cheese (only full fat)
- Seeds –pumpkin, sunflower, flax, chia, etc.
- Avocados – you only need a little sea salt for an awesome high-fiber snack
- Cocoa nibs – a quick, great, sugarless option to chocolate bars
- Seaweed
- A stevia sweetened chocolate (like ChocoPerfection or Lily's) or any Dark chocolate (above 75%)
- Jerky
- String cheese

Chapter 9. Ketogenic Diet Success Tips
Tips and Tricks for Maintaining the Diet

Starting a ketogenic diet

If you're following the standard American diet, a diet where all your calories come from carbohydrates then starting a keto diet will be your best bet. There are two choices for you to choose from which are the cold turkey or eliminating carbohydrates from your diet and increasing fat intake to increase your macronutrients ratios. When cold turkey you will have an unpleasant experience with carbohydrate removal symptoms so the best bet will be eliminating it slowly from your diet.

Carbohydrate guides

This is a guide that will be helpful for you as you are starting out with a ketogenic diet. Carbohydrate guides are books provided for the novice; it enumerates foods and their Carbohydrate content as well as their calorie, protein and fat content. Some even have each category like high carbohydrate, medium, and low carbohydrate lists. There are some mobile apps that have Carbohydrate guides too.

Well, any method you will like to use is up to you, but you should always have your Carbohydrate guides handy when on a shopping spree. You should always recheck to be sure about the food you can consume on the diet and the one that isn't allowed. So go ahead with it for now because as you get acquainted with the guide, you get used to it and know exactly the food to buy so you have nothing to worry about. If you're always unsure about your purchases it's pertinent that you go with your guide all the time.

Prepare your kitchen

When once you have opted to start the ketogenic diet you have to also prepare your kitchen for these changes. Here you have two things to do. One you need to do away with food that is not in accordance with the keto diet. Go through places like your pantry and refrigerator and remove all the off-plan foods that would never fit into your diet plan. Ensure that you check the labels on your spices and even dried herbs. This is to be sure that these herbs don't contain sugar and other artificial ingredients that don't belong in your keto diet, You don't know what to do, well I will tell you. If you have unopened items that are against your diet, you can donate to a local food vendor or give it to a friend, then for the already opened one,s you can trash them or still give it to whoever needs it. But if you don't like that idea just packed all the non-plan foods to one side of the pantry and securely lock them up in such a way you will hardly see them, so as to avoid seeing them and wanting to indulge in them. Leave all ketogenic approved foods in a separate space too and zero your mind to only get to the ketogenic side only. All of this stress is to help you separate what you can eat from what you can't.

Lastly, stock up your home with only what you really need and try to always have a healthy option of food to eat to avoid eating whatever you lay your hands on

Ease into it

When you are thrilled to go on a new eating routine, it is entirely enticing to leap right in; however, your body will be grateful to you if you gradually adopt the ketogenic diet. By so doing, you will decrease the extent to which you may exhibit any of the "keto flu" side effects that you may very well experience and as such make the evolution less problematic. Give yourself three weeks to a month from the day that you make up your mind to adopt a ketogenic diet to the day you really begin it 100 percent.

In the first week of starting the ketogenic diet, let go of every single sugary drink. Examples of such drinks are soft drinks, lemonade, sweetened tea, and flavored drinking waters. In a situation where you add sugar to your coffee, downsize- rather than use two teaspoons, make use of just one. Following a full week of this, do away with all sweets and sugary snacks from the food you consume, including candy cookies, cakes, muffins, chocolates, as well as ice cream. Get used to not having any dessert after supper. You need to prepare your body to quit wanting desserts, and one approach to do this is to remove them totally, particularly while you're changing to a ketogenic diet. During the second week, remove starchy carbohydrates, for example, pasta, pizza, bread, crackers, rolls, and potatoes. Now, you may have begun to get more fit.

By the start of week 2, you'll be all set to truly start up your ketogenic diet. It is at this point that you begin to monitor your macronutrients to ensure you are not going beyond the right proportions. Placing a limit on carbohydrates is essential, yet it's by all account not the only aim; ensure you're likewise eating a lot of fat and reasonable measures of protein.

Remain hydrated and replenish electrolytes

Remaining hydrated is at all times vital; however, it's particularly important when you are beginning a ketogenic diet. It's not just about drinking water; you likewise need to top off your electrolytes. When you begin a ketogenic diet, the first thing is that you lose water, which takes electrolytes like sodium and potassium with it. Make it a goal to drink what could be compared to at least half your body weight in ounces. For instance, if your weight is 180 pounds, you'll need to drink nothing below 90 ounces of water each day.

You can top off your electrolytes by taking a cup of homemade broth each day, adding salt to your nourishment, and drinking waters that are improved with electrolytes. Simply ensure that the improved waters are unflavored, as the enhanced waters regularly contain plenty of sugar and other ingredients that are non-natural.

Planning Meals for Long-Term Success

To record a long-lasting success while on a ketogenic diet, it is important to develop a meal plan. "When you fail to plan, you plan to fail," is a common statement usually credited to Benjamin Franklin. This statement is correct. The most ideal approach to guarantee achievement is to plan your meals for each and every week ahead of time and ensure that you have ketogenic-approved snacks available.

Meal planning

Pick a night each week and list out all that you will eat the whole week. Plan your meals and dinners and afterward put together a shopping list for what you'll require so as to effect these meals and snacks. You may decide to make the day you plan your meals, be the same day you do your grocery shopping also. Get all that you need at once and afterward don't drift from your plan.

Meal prep

As long as you know what you will be eating every day of the week, it is possible that you choose to prepare every dish separately, or you may choose that putting in a couple of hours preparing your dishes is more reasonable for you. In the event that you pick the last option, pick a day in the week when you don't have some other responsibilities and put in a couple of hours in the kitchen set up your meals for the whole week. You can make a pie, a few casseroles that are ketogenic-accommodating dishes, and a large pot of soup. Each meal should then be divided into separate to-go containers then stored in the fridge with the goal that they're all set when you are.

Be prepared

When you're on a specific eating routine, for example, the ketogenic one, there is extremely no such thing as convenience dishes. You must be all set at every point in time. You may need to take meals and snacks along wherever you go, but it is only a little price to pay for the feeling you will get. Put together a lunch each day and keep snacks that are nonperishable, such as fat bombs, coconut shavings, nuts, and seeds in your vehicle, in your work desk in your office, and in your purse or suitcase.

Try not to make it complicated

It's enticing to desire to make complex meal setups that feature yet another gourmet entrée every night, except for a great many people, that is simply not practical. You need to ensure that your new eating routine plan can fit into your way of life; else you won't most likely keep to it. Keep things easy by eating a similar thing for breakfast three days in each and making use of food scraps from supper for the following day's lunch. You can choose to double the recipe or even triple it, to prepare dishes in mass and afterward put it in the freezer to preserve for a day when you don't have the spare time to cook.

Beginning another eating regimen isn't simple; it takes devotion and readiness. You'll need to do some adjusting and reworking to make sense of what works for you; however, once you understand it, it will turn out to be second nature.

Chapter 10. FAQ

Is a keto diet safe?

Normally, a keto diet is very harmless. Nonetheless, in the three circumstances stated below, you may require additional readiness or adjustment:
- Are you taking drugs for diabetes, for example, insulin?
- Are you taking drugs for hypertension?
- Are you breastfeeding?

In case you're not in one of these circumstances, you will most definitely do alright on a keto diet, without requiring any exceptional changes.

Take note that there are legends and misunderstandings about keto, which scares both kids and adults.

What Signals Will You See To Help You Know That Your Body Has Entered Ketosis?

Any of the following signs may show that you are in ketosis:
- Decreased craving and higher energy levels.
- Increased thirst and pee.
- "Keto breath," which might be more obvious to others than to yourself.
- Dry mouth or a metallic flavor for your mouth.

Past these signs and signals, you can calculate your level of ketosis, by making use of any one of these three strategies:
- Urine strips
- Breath analyzers
- Blood meters

Is a Keto Diet Harmless for the Kidneys?
Truly. Individuals regularly wonder about this, due to the conviction that an eating routine high in protein could be hurtful for the kidneys. Be that as it may, this fear is just founded on two mistaken assumptions:
- A keto diet is high in fat, not protein.
- People with normal functioning kidney handle too much protein just fine.

As such, there is no reason to stress. Truth be told, a keto diet may even be helpful of your kidneys, particularly in the event that you have diabetes.

Will I Be Able to Eat Dairy and Nuts on Keto?
Truly, if your body endures them well.

The issue with nuts and dairy is that they are trigger foods for some individuals, and not every person measures and tracks them accurately, which can cause a slow rate of weight loss.

Furthermore, a few people don't process them so well, which can even lead to inflammation and water retention.

In the event that you are as of now battling with a difficulty in weight reduction, make an effort to limit nuts and dairy for a few weeks to check whether that makes a difference. After that, you can gradually introduce them to your body and see how your body responds.

How Do I Know If I'm in Ketosis? Do I Need to Measure Ketones?
You don't have to gauge ketones, yet a few people do. Here are a few signs that you're in ketosis:
- losing a great deal of water weight in one or two days – 5 to 10 pounds is normal
- diminished or increased energy
- lower craving

- a sweet or metallic flavor in your mouth or a fruity keto breath.

If you need to know with sureness whether or not you have entered into Ketosis, ensure that you observe yourself to take note of all the above-mentioned ways to measure levels of ketone.

On a Ketogenic Diet, is it Necessary That I Monitor my Calories and Macros?

Yes, particularly at the start, until you become accustomed to it. The issue with carbs is that they're all over the place and that even little amounts rapidly add up.

The most ideal way to ensure you are maintaining under 20-25 g net carbs daily is by simply taking measurements and closely monitoring what you're eating.

For this purpose, it is required that you get a food scale and make use of a tracking application where you record what you're eating using a keto diet application.

Concerning calories, so as to lose weight, you have to make a caloric shortfall, as such you should find out what your calories for maintenance are, and after that subtract 15% to 25% from that number, to get your caloric aim.

Greater shortfalls will probably cause an increasingly fast weight reduction which is not so much sustainable but rather harder to keep up. With a little deficiency, you'll possibly get more fit at a slower rate; however, it will be less demanding for your body (and mind).

Numerous individuals choose to do what is regularly called "lazy keto" when they achieve their objective weight, that is, eat keto meals without essentially tracking them, or tracking from time to time to see where they stand regarding macros and calories. This is suggested just on the off chance that you've achieved your objective weight and now have loads ketogenic diet experience.

Low Carb and Keto, are they the same?
Keto is a sort of a low-carb diet. Low-carb is an unclearly explained term that can be applied to just about any eating regimen where carbs are restricted, and keto is one of the very strict kinds of low-carb. Low-carb can be defined as anything from 20-25 g net carbs daily (strict keto) to about 100-120 net carbs every day.

Are Carbs Needed For Body Functioning?
Although it is true that your body, and particularly your brain, need some carbs to work, there are two interesting points:
- The required quantity is extremely little.
- Your body can create the needed glucose by means of a procedure called gluconeogenesis (GNG). That is the reason the human body can even deal with a zero-carb kind of eating regimen.

Isn't All This Fat Unhealthy?
To put it plainly, the answer is no. It is possible you will be eating a lot more fat than you used to, but fat ought not to be dreaded, and saturated fat really has its place in a heart-healthy eating routine.

You ought to steer clear of highly processes fats, for example, canola oil or soybean oil, just as trans-fats.

In the event that you adhere to the fat from meat and eggs, just as to different sorts of healthy fats, for example, avocado oil, coconut oil, and olive oil, you do not have anything to fear.

With respect to cholesterol, the association between cholesterol in your diet and the cholesterol in your blood has for some time now been disproven – a higher percentage of the cholesterol in your body is produced by your body, and not absorbed from meals.

I'm Vegan/Vegetarian. Would I Still be Able to do Keto?

Certainly. Although one of the primary sources of a keto diet is meat, there are a lot of options that you could pick from and make it work for you in case you are a veggie lover or vegan.

I Started Doing Keto Only a Few Days Ago. Why Am I Feeling So Exhausted and Weak?

What you are having is called keto flu. This isn't strange, particularly on the off chance that it is your first time ever doing keto, and it will go in a few days.

Your body is adjusting to making use of fat for fuel rather than carbs, which is a lot of changes, so you should simply give it some time, ensure you remain hydrated, and that your electrolytes are within proper limits.

The keto flu is the initial part of a much longer process regularly called "fat adaptation," in which your body changes gears and turns out to be better suited in making use of fat as its essential fuel source. The keto flu, in any case, more often than not lasts for a lesser period, around 2-3 days to seven days.

How Long Does It Take to Get Into Ketosis?

It ordinarily takes between 2-4 days to get into ketosis, but this depends upon your exercises level and digestion. Individuals with more insulin resistance (for example individuals with type 2 diabetes) normally take longer, while youthful and lean individuals usually get into ketosis unquestionably more rapidly.

How Long Does It Take to be Fat-Adapted?

It could rake about three weeks to a month and a half or more of being in ketosis.

Why Am I Not in Ketosis?

The two commonest explanations behind not entering ketosis are;
- Too much protein
- Too many carbs

Kindly note that the quantities that individuals endure while remaining in ketosis are individual, contrasting from individual to individual.

In the Case of High Cholesterol, is a Ketogenic Diet Safe?

The cholesterol profile will, in general, be better on a keto diet, bringing down triglycerides and raising the good HDL cholesterol.

Notwithstanding, a little minority of individuals may finish up with very high all out cholesterol. Regardless of whether this is harmful or harmless is under discussion- there aren't any quality investigations to decide the appropriate response. Be that as it may, should you be among the few cases where cholesterol levels shoot up, for example above 400, you might need to find a way to decrease so as to remain on the safer side.

Would I Be Able to Have Organic Products on a Keto Diet?

In spite of the fact that natural products- fruits- are regularly viewed as healthy, in reality, they contain a very high carbs and sugar content, unlike that which is seen in vegetables that are free from starch. As such, with regards to ketone based diets, a lot of fruits should be avoided.

In any case, certain types of berries are excluded and can be consumed in little quantities. The best options are blackberries, raspberries, and strawberries, which give 5-6 grams of carb per 100 grams (3½ ounces).

A lot of other fruits– including blueberries – contain in them up to double or triple this measure of carbs, as shown in this book for the best and worst fruits depending on the carb content.

Remember that berries don't give any supplements that can't be found in vegetables and different other foods with lower carb levels, so they are altogether non-compulsory on a keto diet. Truth be told, in the event that you are very resistant to insulin, it may be more ideal for you not to have them.

Would I Be Able to Have Dairy on Keto?

Dairy is nutritious, and it can be a part of a keto diet in many instances. Be that as it may, regardless of whether consume dairy or not may rely upon your wellbeing objectives, alongside your own reaction to it.

For example, although the consumption of dairy at a higher level has been connected to fat loss as well as lower diabetes risk in a few investigations, it has likewise been found to raise insulin levels. Truly, a few people discovered reducing intake level of dairy helps with weight reduction.

It's additionally vital to steer clear from high-carb alternatives regularly thought to be "healthy," for example, milk and yogurt that have no fat in them. Rather, let your focus be these high-fat options, ideally from naturally raised animals:

- Cream
- Sour cream
- Cream cheddar
- Cheese
- Plain whole-milk yogurt, Greek yogurt, or kefir

What Differentiates a Low-carb Diet from a Keto Diet?

Keto is an extremely strict low-carb diet, which additionally puts significantly more stress on regulating protein consumption, and depending essentially on fat to supply energy requirements.

A standard strict low-carb diet will probably put a lot of people in ketosis at any rate. In any case, a keto diet changes things significantly to ensure it's working and, as desired, get a lot more in-depth into ketosis whenever.

Keto could be referred to as a low-carb diet, but one that is extra-strict.

To Accelerate the Loss of Weight Should I Target High Ketone Levels?

The response to this is a Yes and no. Consuming fewer carbs, less protein and practicing irregular fasting surely advances weight reduction, while bringing down insulin and raising ketone levels.

In any case, adding more fat, or supplementing with MCT oil, or drinking "exogenous" ketone supplements does not improve weight reduction. These techniques, in reality, reduce the rate at which weight is lost, by giving other fuel to be utilized as opposed to burning fat in the body.

On the off chance that you need to get thinner, just make use of these techniques – MCT (Medium-Chain Triglycerides) oil or ketones that happen to be exogenous – whenever you are starving, or for the purpose of performance (not in any way connected to weight reduction).

At what time would it be advisable for you to test ketone levels?

It is especially good to measure ketone levels at about the same time daily for the purpose of comparison. Taking the ketone level measurement every morning before breakfast makes it a lot less difficult to make comparisons with measurements taken daily.

In any case, morning numbers are more often than not among the most minimal of the day, while evening numbers tend to be higher. So if for reasons unknown you need amazingly high numbers, measure in the nights. Know that your ketone levels don't recognize the difference between utilization of fat contained in your diet and fat stored in your body

Is Keto Harmless During Pregnancy?

In light of the encounters of people who have done it as well as the doctors who have treated patients using a keto diet while pregnant, the keto diet during pregnancy seems to be safe. It might likewise be exceptionally useful if a case of gestational diabetes does arise.

Notwithstanding, there are no scientific investigations regarding the matter, so there is an absence of precise knowledge. It is probably wise to be cautious and go for an increasingly moderate low-carb diet while pregnant, except if there are vital medical advantages of doing a keto diet in your particular case.

While on a Ketogenic Diet, Am I Permitted to Have Cheat Meals?

Cheating is not a good idea. It will cause you to discontinue ketosis and influence your process of fat adjustment. It will only give rise to carb longings and might promote an increase in weight after consumption of cheat meals.

We are all just human, and we do commit errors. On the off chance that this occurs, pardon yourself and proceed. Just begin eating keto again directly after the cheat feast.

On Keto is it Possible That I Lose Muscle Mass? Would I be able to Build More Muscle On Keto?

In case you're eating adequate protein, there would not be cause for you to lose muscle mass – on the other hand, keto is muscle saving. Furthermore, you can likewise gain more muscle (given that you're doing some sort of resistance exercise and eating right).

Remember that reducing weight and building muscle all at once is not easy, albeit unquestionably possible, particularly for individuals who just started exercising.

If I begin Keto, Will my Athletic Performance go Downhill?

At the start, it just might. Amid the adjustment stage, numerous individuals experience reduction in performance, be it in their perseverance, power or explosive force.

This will go away with time, given that you provide your body with enough time to adjust and that you are also supplementing the much-needed electrolytes (they're fundamental for everybody, except considerably more so for individuals that are more active).

Are Supplements Necessary for me During Keto?

Electrolytes, for example, magnesium and sodium, have to be supplemented. In addition, you need to ensure you're getting enough potassium from your nourishment.

Aside from that, numerous individuals choose to supplement with MCT oil or powder, creatine, fish oil, etc. These supplements are by no means required; however, a few of the supplements may just be advantageous for you.

I'm Craving Carbs/Sweets, What Should I Do?

This is totally a normal feeling, and numerous individuals experience a period where they hunger for carbs. This will leave with time, so the most critical thing is simply to not lose patience.

There are a couple of things you can do in case you are longing for carbs, for example,

- stay very much hydrated
- on your first few days on the keto diet, eat until you are satisfied
- prepare a keto dessert for yourself.

I Have Entered Ketosis and Not Losing Weight. What am I to do?

In case your weight is not reducing after over two weeks to three weeks, this implies you have reached a setback (keto plateau). There are a couple of things you could do to assist you with that:

- ensure you are eating under your maintenance calories
- ensure you are tracking everything that you're consuming
- ensure that you are keeping your electrolytes under control
- try limiting cheese and nuts to check whether that makes a difference
- track your progress using not only your scale but also by taking progress photographs and measures (hips, waist, thighs, for instance) – if you have begun working out, it is possible that you are gaining muscle mass while at the same time losing fat
- patiently let time pass

Weight reduction is not linear – the scale will once in a while go up, or won't move for a considerable length of time or weeks. You may even be gaining a couple of pounds during the menstrual cycle, and it's totally normal. The most vital thing is to watch out for the common trend to be consistent.

Am I in Need of Exogenous Ketones?
Simply put, no. Exogenous ketones do have a few advantages; however, they are not essential on keto.

In Conjunction with Keto, What are the Other Things that I Can Do to Better my Health?
There are various things you can do to enhance your wellbeing, and you can join them with keto very effectively, depending on the objective of your keto diet. Here are a few thoughts:
- Exercise: exercise includes resistance training, cardio exercise, high-intensity interval training (HIIT), or a blend of those. Discover a sport that you really do like and that it is possible for you to be consistent with over a long time period. Exercise ought to be fun and not feel like a task, and consistency is vital.
- Be active in your everyday life: walk more, discover a hobby that has a physical component to it, take the stairs rather than the elevator. There are a lot of approaches to sneak in some physical activity into your life.
- Ensure that you are getting enough sleep and rest: exercise and diet are essential; however, in case you're not getting enough sleep, your results will suffer. Concerning rest, in case you're exceptionally physically active, ensure your body has sufficient resting time. Going to the gym on a daily basis may prompt fatigue and trauma. Get no less than 1 or 2 days of the week off to rest.
- Intermittent fasting (IF): IF is a great system for weight

reduction and for enhancing your general wellbeing.

In general, in case you're keen on enhancing your wellbeing, your goal should be; consuming healthy meals, being more active, and also providing yourself with the right amount of rest. If it so happens that you are consistent, before long, you will begin seeing changes.

Will I Gain All The Lost Weight Back If I Choose To Stop My Keto Diet?

Not at all, given that you don't return to the harmful routine that made you put on the weight to start with.

You ought not to see keto as some kind of fast solution, or fad diet that you do for a period of about 2-3 months and afterward put it out of your mind.

Regardless of whether you choose to adopt a moderate approach to carbs once you achieve your objective weight, you should ensure that you're ready to stick to eating well and not to eat too much all the time.

So as to keep the weight off, you have to ensure you have really changed your way of life and not simply "gone on a diet" to then return to eating unhealthy meals.

If you choose to reintroduce carbs after achieving your objective weight, we suggest doing it gradually and watching out for how your body responds to them; there are a lot of other great solutions that are not so limiting, for example, low-carb, paleo, primal, etc.

If you choose to never do keto again, you will put back on some water weight (often between 5 to 10 pounds) – this isn't fat, and you don't have anything to fear. If you need to ward off the fat, however, you should be sensible and watch that your calories are under control.

Would I be able to Do Keto Long Term?

To this, the answer is yes, and several individuals do. Simply keep to keto if you feel best on it.

How long can someone be on a keto diet?

For whatever length of time, you enjoy it and need to.

Conclusion

I really hope you have discovered this book in great health, and I wish you continuous progress on your low carb diet. Kindly refer back to this book anytime you find yourself retreating back to the old unhealthy way of life, it will return you to the path of success.

Your work is not finished after the 28-day cycle has been completed. Never forget that 'weight is managed, not cured.'

After you have maintained a low carb diet for some time, you will start to notice the approximate place you ought to be at in your everyday 'net carbs' to be capable of maintaining your weight loss easily for life.

I highly advise that you keep data that is accurate on your everyday food intake.

Stefano Villa

Sources

1-4 [online] Available at: https://www.coursehero.com/file/p2gk19t/Spinach-Salad-4-Cups-Spinach-4-Tbsp -Olive-Oil-3-Tbsp -Leftover-Meat-624-Calories/ [Accessed 24 Feb. 2019].

5 Keto Bootstrap. (2019). Almond Lemon Sandwich Cakes Keto Recipe. [online] Available at: https://ketobootstrap.com/recipe/almond-lemon-sandwich-cakes [Accessed 25 Feb. 2019].

6 Cdn.ruled.me. (2019). [online] Available at: https://cdn.ruled.me/wp-content/uploads/2014/02/almondlemoncakes1.jpg [Accessed 25 Feb. 2019].

7 Burger, L. (2019). Inside Out Bacon Burger | Ruled Me. [online] Ruled Me. Available at: https://www.ruled.me/inside-out-bacon-burger/ [Accessed 25 Feb. 2019].

8 Cdn.ruled.me. (2019). [online] Available at: https://cdn.ruled.me/wp-content/uploads/2014/03/baconburger.jpg [Accessed 25 Feb. 2019].

9 Beefandlambni.com. (2019). [online] Available at: https://www.beefandlambni.com/siteFiles/resources/MozzarellaMeatballswithtomatoandbacon1109x627.jpg [Accessed 25 Feb. 2019].

10 Meatballs, B. (2019). Bacon & Mozzarella Meatballs | Ruled Me. [online] Ruled Me. Available at:

https://www.ruled.me/bacon-mozzarella-meatballs/ [Accessed 25 Feb. 2019].

11   Peas, B. (2019). Bacon Infused Sugar Snap Peas. [online] MealPlannerPro.com. Available at: https://mealplannerpro.com/member-recipes/Bacon-Infused-Sugar-Snap-Peas-628180 [Accessed 25 Feb. 2019].

12   Chicken, S. (2019). Simple Keto BBQ Pulled Chicken. [online] MealPlannerPro.com. Available at: https://mealplannerpro.com/member-recipes/Simple-Keto-BBQ-Pulled-Chicken-404960 [Accessed 5 Mar. 2019].

13   Cmt.azureedge.net. (2019). [online] Available at: https://cmt.azureedge.net/media/buffalo-chicken-strips-20180102151135548500en0f.jpg [Accessed 25 Feb. 2019].

14   Strips, S. (2019). Superbowl Sunday Buffalo Strips | Ruled Me. [online] Ruled Me. Available at: https://www.ruled.me/superbowl-sunday-buffalo-strips/ [Accessed 25 Feb. 2019].

15   Ruled Me. (2019). Perfect Cup of Ketoproof Coffee | Ruled Me. [online] Available at: https://www.ruled.me/ketoproof-coffee/ [Accessed 5 Mar. 2019].

16   Cake, C. (2019). Chai Spice Keto Mug Cake | Ruled Me. [online] Ruled Me. Available at: https://www.ruled.me/chai-spice-keto-mug-cake/ [Accessed 25 Feb. 2019].

17   Explosion, C. (2019). Cheddar Bacon Explosion |

Ruled Me. [online] Ruled Me. Available at: https://www.ruled.me/cheddar-bacon-explosion/ [Accessed 25 Feb. 2019].

18   Meatballs, C. (2019). Chorizo & Cheddar Cheese Meatballs | Ruled Me. [online] Ruled Me. Available at: https://www.ruled.me/chorizo-cheddar-cheese-meatballs/ [Accessed 25 Feb. 2019].

19   Media.eggs.ca. (2019). [online] Available at: https://media.eggs.ca/assets/RecipePhotos/_resampled/FillWyIxMjgwIiwiNzIwIl0/Scrambled-Eggs-v1.jpg [Accessed 25 Feb. 2019].

20   Anon, (2019). [online] Available at: https://cavemanketo.com/wp-content/uploads/2012/02/IMG_20120215_185516-660x330.jpg [Accessed 25 Feb. 2019].

21   Assets.bonappetit.com. (2019). [online] Available at: https://assets.bonappetit.com/photos/57ae4b1153e63daf11a4e4d7/16:9/w_1280,c_limit/chicken-roulade.jpg [Accessed 25 Feb. 2019].

22   The Pioneer Woman. (2019). Buffalo Chicken Sliders. [online] Available at: https://thepioneerwoman.com/food-and-friends/buffalo-chicken-sliders/ [Accessed 25 Feb. 2019].

23   Bacon, C. (2019). Bacon, Cheddar and Chive Mug Cake | Ruled Me. [online] Ruled Me. Available at: https://www.ruled.me/bacon-cheddar-chive-mug-cake/ [Accessed 25 Feb. 2019].

24   Meljoulwan.com. (2019). [online] Available at:

https://www.meljoulwan.com/wp-content/uploads/2010/02/beefstew.jpg [Accessed 25 Feb. 2019].

25. Schwartz, S. (2019). Coffee and Wine Beef Stew Recipe | The Nosher. [online] My Jewish Learning. Available at: https://www.myjewishlearning.com/the-nosher/coffee-and-wine-beef-stew-recipe/ [Accessed 25 Feb. 2019].

26. Myfitnesspal.com. (2019). Calorie Chart, Nutrition Facts, Calories in Food | MyFitnessPal | MyFitnessPal.com. [online] Available at: https://www.myfitnesspal.com/food/calories/keto-crispy-curry-rubbed-chicken-thighs-282875976 [Accessed 25 Feb. 2019].

27. Beef, D. (2019). Drunken Five Spice Beef. [online] MealPlannerPro.com. Available at: https://mealplannerpro.com/member-recipes/Drunken-Five-Spice-Beef-905141 [Accessed 25 Feb. 2019].

28. Imstillinbed.files.wordpress.com. (2019). [online] Available at: https://imstillinbed.files.wordpress.com/2015/06/cheesy-frittata-muffins.jpg [Accessed 25 Feb. 2019].

29. Eat This Much, I. (2019). Eat This Much, your personal diet assistant. [online] Eat This Much. Available at: https://www.eatthismuch.com/recipe/nutrition/cheesy-frittata-muffins,364652/ [Accessed 25 Feb. 2019].

30 OneEarthHealth. (2019). Fried Queso Fresco. [online] Available at: https://oneearthhealth.com/blogs/keto-recipes/fried-queso-fresco [Accessed 25 Feb. 2019].

31 OneEarthHealth. (2019). Lemon & Rosemary Roasted Chicken Thighs. [online] Available at: https://oneearthhealth.com/blogs/keto-recipes/lemon-rosemary-roasted-chicken-thighs [Accessed 25 Feb. 2019].

32 Eat This Much, I. (2019). Eat This Much, your personal diet assistant. [online] Eat This Much. Available at: https://www.eatthismuch.com/recipe/nutrition/keto-szechuan-chicken,955690/ [Accessed 25 Feb. 2019].

33 KD Recipes. (2019). Modified Not Your Caveman's Chili. [online] Available at: https://kdrecipesblog.wordpress.com/2017/09/08/modified-not-your-Caveman's-chili/ [Accessed 25 Feb. 2019].

34 OneEarthHealth. (2019). Omnivore Burger with Creamed Spinach and Roasted Almonds. [online] Available at: https://oneearthhealth.com/blogs/keto-recipes/omnivore-burger-with-creamed-spinach-and-roasted-almonds [Accessed 25 Feb. 2019].

35 Tenderloin, B. (2019). Bacon Wrapped Pork Tenderloin | Ruled Me. [online] Ruled Me. Available at: https://www.ruled.me/bacon-wrapped-pork-tenderloin/ [Accessed 25 Feb. 2019].

36   Salad, R. (2019). Red Pepper Spinach Salad | Ruled Me. [online] Ruled Me. Available at: https://www.ruled.me/red-pepper-spinach-salad/ [Accessed 25 Feb. 2019].

37   Keto Carlo. (2019). ROASTED PECAN GREEN BEANS. [online] Available at: https://www.ketocarlo.com/roasted-pecan-green-beans.html [Accessed 25 Feb. 2019].

38   Keto Carlo. (2019). SHRIMP & CAULIFLOWER CURRY. [online] Available at: https://www.ketocarlo.com/shrimp--cauliflower-curry.html [Accessed 25 Feb. 2019].

39   Keto Carlo. (2019). KETO SNICKERDOODLE COOKIES. [online] Available at: https://www.ketocarlo.com/keto-snickerdoodle-cookies.html [Accessed 25 Feb. 2019].

40   Keto Carlo. (2019). LOW CARB SPICE CAKES. [online] Available at: https://www.ketocarlo.com/low-carb-spice-cakes.html [Accessed 25 Feb. 2019].

41   Fry, C. (2019). Chicken and Bacon Sausage Stir Fry | Ruled Me. [online] Ruled Me. Available at: https://www.ruled.me/chicken-bacon-sausage-stir-fry/ [Accessed 25 Feb. 2019].

42   Tartlets, L. (2019). Low Carb Taco Tartlets | Ruled Me. [online] Ruled Me. Available at: https://www.ruled.me/low-carb-taco-tartlets/ [Accessed 25 Feb. 2019].

43   Allrecipes. (2019). Thai Peanut Chicken Recipe.

[online] Available at: https://www.allrecipes.com/recipe/50658/thai-peanut-chicken/ [Accessed 25 Feb. 2019].

44 Anon, (2019). [online] Available at: http://sugarcrafter.net/2011/11/03/vanilla-latte-cookies/ [Accessed 25 Feb. 2019].

45 Medley, D. (2019). Delicious Vegetable Medley | Ruled Me. [online] Ruled Me. Available at: https://www.ruled.me/delicious-vegetable-medley/ [Accessed 5 Mar. 2019].

46 Primaltoad.com. (2019). Low Carb Chocolate Almond Smoothie – Primal Toad. [online] Available at: https://primaltoad.com/low-carb-chocolate-almond-smoothie/ [Accessed 5 Mar. 2019].

47 Liv Breathe Keto. (2019). Pumpkin Pie Protein Shake – Liv Breathe Keto. [online] Available at: https://livbreatheketo.com/pumpkin-pie-protein-shake/ [Accessed 5 Mar. 2019].

48 Simple Green Smoothies. (2019). The BEST Green Smoothie Recipe Ever | Simple Green Smoothies. [online] Available at: https://simplegreensmoothies.com/recipes/beginners-luck-green-smoothie [Accessed 5 Mar. 2019].

49 (2019). Keto Green Smoothie - 4g net carbs - Ditch The Carbs. [online] Ditch The Carbs. Available at: https://www.ditchthecarbs.com/keto-green-smoothie/ [Accessed 5 Mar. 2019].

50 (2019). Hass Avocado Honeydew Smoothie Recipe. [online] Hispanic Kitchen. Available at:

https://hispanickitchen.com/recipes/hass-avocado-honeydew-smoothie-recipe/ [Accessed 5 Mar. 2019].

51   Lindsey Janeiro, C. (2019). Honeydew Avocado Kale Smoothie | Nutrition to Fit. [online] Nutrition to Fit. Available at: https://nutritiontofit.com/honeydew-avocado-kale-smoothie/ [Accessed 5 Mar. 2019].

52   Magary, V. (2019). How To Make A Green Smoothie / Ultimate Paleo Guide. [online] Ultimate Paleo Guide. Available at: https://ultimatepaleoguide.com/make-green-smoothie/ [Accessed 5 Mar. 2019].

53   Raspberry Avocado Smoothie - Dairy Free. (2019). [online] Low Carb Yum. Available at: https://lowcarbyum.com/raspberry-avocado-smoothie-low-carb/ [Accessed 5 Mar. 2019].

54   Smoothie, R. and Smoothie, R. (2019). Raspberry and Avocado Smoothie | Nadia Lim. [online] Nadia Lim. Available at: https://nadialim.com/recipe/raspberry-avocado-smoothie/ [Accessed 5 Mar. 2019].

55   IdealFit. (2019). Triple Green Smoothie | IdealFit. [online] Available at: https://www.idealfit.com/blog/triple-green-smoothie/ [Accessed 5 Mar. 2019].

56   Foodnetwork.com. (2019). Best Almond Milk And Berry Smoothie recipes. [online] Available at: https://www.foodnetwork.com/recipes/melissa-darabian/almond-milk-and-berry-smoothie-recipe-1960870 [Accessed 5 Mar. 2019].

57 Kale and Brazil Nut Smoothie, (2019). [online] Available at: https://www.kroger.com/r/kale-brazil-nut-smoothie-recipe/175389 [Accessed 5 Mar. 2019].

58 Cucumber Spinach Smoothie (2019) | Ruled Me. [online] Ruled Me. Available at: https://www.ruled.me/cucumber-spinach-smoothie/ [Accessed 5 Mar. 2019].

59 Banana Cashew Butter Chia Seed Smoothie - Jar Of Lemons. [online] Jar Of Lemons. Available at: https://www.jaroflemons.com/banana-cashew-butter-chia-seed-smoothie/ [Accessed 5 Mar. 2019].

60 Chai Spiced Cashew Butter & Froothie Optimum 9400 Review - Domestic Gothess. [online] Available at: https://domesticgothess.com/blog/2018/01/24/chai-spiced-cashew-butter/ [Accessed 5 Mar. 2019].

61 Oaxaca Chocolate Banana Smoothie Recipe - Cookie and Kate. [online] Cookie and Kate. Available at: https://cookieandkate.com/2013/oaxaca-chocolate-banana-smoothie/ [Accessed 5 Mar. 2019].

62 Day, R. (2019). Coconut-Orange Smoothie. [online] Rachael Ray Every Day. Available at: https://www.rachaelraymag.com/recipe/coconut-orange-smoothie [Accessed 5 Mar. 2019].

63 Stews, S., Appetizers, S., Desserts, C., Bars, C., Me, A., Policy, P., Me, W., (thespicetrain.com), n. and Eggs, A. (2019). Creamy Orange Coconut Smoothie | Occasionally Eggs. [online] Occasionally Eggs.

Available at: https://www.occasionallyeggs.com/creamy-orange-coconut-smoothie/ [Accessed 5 Mar. 2019].

64   Tri-Wellness. (2019). Banana Berry Lettuce Smoothie - Tri-Wellness. [online] Available at: https://lisashanken.com/recipe/banana-berry-lettuce-smoothie/ [Accessed 5 Mar. 2019].

65   Banana, G. (2019). Green Smoothie: Romaine Lettuce & Banana Recipe. [online] SparkRecipes. Available at: https://recipes.sparkpeople.com/recipe-detail.asp?recipe=1581664 [Accessed 5 Mar. 2019].

66   Creme De La Crumb. (2019). Banana Nut Smoothie Bowl | Creme De La Crumb. [online] Available at: https://www.lecremedelacrumb.com/banana-nut-smoothie-bowl/ [Accessed 5 Mar. 2019].

Printed in Great Britain
by Amazon